FELL IN HER HANDS

Fell in Her Hands

Ruth Lauer-Manenti

Lantern Books ● New York
A Division of Booklight Inc.

2016

Lantern Books

128 Second Place

Brooklyn, NY 11231

www.lanternbooks.com

Printed in the United States of America

Names: Lauer Manenti, Ruth, author. | Pataänjali. Yogasåutra. English.
Title: Fell in her hands : a retelling of the Yoga Sutra of Patanjali / Ruth
Lauer Manenti.
Description: New York : Lantern Books, 2016.
Identifiers: LCCN 2015036519| ISBN 9781590565315 (pbk. : alk. paper) | ISBN
9781590565322 (ebook)
Subjects: LCSH: Yoga—Early works to 1800.
Classification: LCC B132.Y6 L38 2016 | DDC 181/.452—dc23
LC record available at http://lccn.loc.gov/2015036519

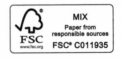

The first thing to do is to find a sacred place to live.
Ma Bhaskarananda

For Fernanda Manenti

CONTENTS

Introduction xi

Book I: Absorption.. I
Book II: Practice 47
Book III: Ash 107
Book IV: The Rain Cloud 139
The Yoga Sutra of Patanjali 183

Acknowledgments 213

About the Author
About the Publisher

INTRODUCTION

The *Yoga Sutra* is attributed to an enlightened being named Maharishi Patanjali, who lived some time between 400 BCE and 400 CE. There are various accounts about his birth. One is that he fell (*pat*) from heaven into the palms (*anjali*) of a woman who was praying to have a child. He appeared in the form of a snake, later described as having one thousand heads, each head representing a *pundit*, or spiritual teacher, yet all connected to one body or source/origin of knowledge. The fact that Maharishi (the great seer) first appeared as a snake may seem strange or even unbelievable to some, but these ideas are meant to be pondered for meaning's sake rather than argued over for proof. When one looks at the ways of a snake, and animals in general, one can certainly find a lot of wisdom.

The *Yoga Sutra* is made up of four books with approximately 196 sutras in toto, which distill the teachings and ideas on yoga that were already in the *Upanishads*, composed centuries earlier. Within the sutras lies the essence of yoga philosophy and practice. The word *sutra* means "thread," or that which stitches together, though often hidden or only visible from the back, as in under a hem. The text is called the *Yoga Sutra*, implying that all the sutras stitched together make one sutra, such that each sutra relates to all that comes before and after, for a full comprehension, much like life. The sutras are short and so lend themselves well to memorization and discussion. In the minimal number of words lies an infinite amount of meaning. The text, from book to book, verse to verse, and word to word, is organized in a way that demands deep study and reflection, inspiring multiple readings with a wide range of understandings, and one finds oneself taking the text apart so as to put it back together.

I have wanted to write a commentary and translation on the *Yoga Sutra* for many years, and began composing a book six years ago. I was especially encouraged by the students at the Jivamukti Yoga School in New York City, who have expressed gratitude for the way I teach the *Yoga Sutra* through storytelling. After three years of hard work, I realized that my understanding of the text, both intellectually and experientially, as well as my knowledge of Sanskrit (the original language of the *Yoga Sutra*), was not extensive enough to write a commentary. So I stopped working on the project, thinking I was incapable of writing it in the way it warranted. Then one day, as I was walking down the street, the idea came to me of a female character living in Maharishi Patanjali's world. She would experience the levels of consciousness that he describes, while simultaneously inhabiting my mind.

The result is this book. The story and its characters emerge out of the sutras, with the characters developing and evolving through the various obstacles and challenges that are presented in the *Yoga Sutra*. What I realized while I was writing was the story within the *Yoga Sutra* itself. I decided not to interweave the actual sutras themselves with Clara's story, and instead have placed them at the end for the sake of fluidity, so that one can read through the story or through the translations without interruption.

My humble translations of the sutras are poetic and non-literal, offered in the hopes that the correlation between the sutras and Clara's life give the reader a worthwhile experience. In some cases, the same idea is articulated in different ways to enter into the abstraction of the sutra, and make it more comprehensible. I see it in the same way as you might count to 4. There are several possible means of doing this: $2 + 2$, $1 + 3$, $3 + 1$, but also $5 - 1$. You reach the same result, but do so through many paths. This is how I have shaped my translations and this is the genius of the *Yoga Sutra* of Patanjali. You also might like to read this book alongside the *Yoga Sutra*. There are many excellent versions available, which vary according to translation and commentary. I recommend the *Science of Yoga* by I. K. Taimni and the *Textbook of Yoga Philosophy* by Shri Brahmananda Sarasvati.

The *Yoga Sutra* has provided me with a way of life that has led to the feeling that we animals, plants, and people are not so different from one another; that our consciousness is one, shared, and pure. I am surrounded by wise and kind people. My characters, inspired by the people in my life, have come to similar conclusions. I hope I have not, in any way, offended anyone who might see themselves in one of my characters. My hope was to represent each character as I see them, lovingly. At the same time, all characters are fictions, made up of combinations, histories, and stories of those whom I know and those I don't.

Book I: Absorption

Clara

Clara lived in the present moment in a house with windows on all four sides. She liked each of her four views equally and could see them all at the same time. The trees around the house were old and had grown deep roots. Each tree was unique and she knew the specialties of their uniqueness. She appreciated their diversity, but in essence the trees were all the same to her. She felt herself to be made of the same tree-ness and this was part of her great comfort. The house she lived in at the base of the Pine Forest Mountain was small and unassuming. It was uncluttered, which allowed the natural beauty to be visible, and since there were windows on all four sides, the shafts of sunlight moved through the house from all directions. She observed the dust in these shafts and watched the light move across the walls; as the light moved, she lost track of time. Having lived in an apartment in New York City for twenty-five years, with windows only at one end and a building across the street that blocked most of the light, she was thankful to have windows on all four sides. In the house it was light inside at times and dark at others, depending on the time of day and the cloud cover.

She saw herself in the trees and knew she was not separate from them. She had come to this visualization slowly, as her abilities to concentrate became strong from practices she had been given by her teachers. The spaciousness of her home and its lack of many material objects gave the atmosphere a sacredness where she could sit, attentive and undistracted, and join with the spirit in and around her that she trusted. She looked upon this spirit as a teacher or guide. In her most perspicacious moods she felt this spirit even in a grain of rice or strand of hair.

She liked reading books, particularly those that instructed her on how to live in nature. She loved Hildegard of Bingen, the visionary born in 1098, who combined writing, painting, and music with spiritual healing and became known for her powers involving the application of tinctures made from herbs. Her books *Know the Ways* and *On God's Activities* describe the relationship between the microcosm and the macrocosm of the universe. Her works often focus on patterns of four: the elements (fire, air, water, and earth), the seasons (spring, summer, autumn, winter), the humors (black bile, yellow bile, phlegm, and blood), the zones of the Earth (North, South, East, and West), and the major winds. She understood that the waxing and waning of the moon, the planting of seeds, the bearing and blossoming of fruit, and the birth of an animal or child all came from one interrelated divine cycle. She heard celestial sounds she called the "voice of the Living Light," and composed music from these experiences. She was one of the first women to speak publicly about her visions and interpretations of the scriptures, and was controversial and chastised because of this. When she died, it was said that her sisters saw two streams of light appear in the sky and cross through the room where she was dying. Clara saw threads between the visions of Hildegard and that of the sages from the East that lived far earlier than Hildegard, and felt her life enhanced by her knowledge of their existence.

Clara had discovered from reading Hildegard's books that plants had healing qualities and were medicinal through the trust, praise, and use of them. She collected thoughts in her mind from books she had read by Leo Tolstoy that stated that uprooting a flower with a tough stalk kills the flower, so that even when the flower is in one's hand, one feels empty-handed. The more she learned from her books and teachers and the greater her attunement to her surroundings, the less worried and nervous she was; so that the dark thoughts and negativity that had been in her mind steadily diminished.

Clara's father, Eli, came from Austria. At the age of fifteen, he was forced to leave on account of the impending war. Prior to escaping for America, Eli's family sent ahead all their valuable jewels. These jewels were placed inside a piano, which was shipped to Philadelphia. The jewels stayed for a long time inside the piano, and no one knew they were there except Eli and his family. From this collection of jewels, Eli gave Clara a ring when she turned forty. She loved the ring, thinking about how it had been hidden away for a long time in a musical instrument that had traveled overseas and had once belonged to her great-grandmother. The ring illuminated the poetry of her life and was a symbol of what can't be held, but is expressed through the ring's placement on Clara's middle finger. She liked the way it felt, how it sparkled and became part of her routine, as she took it off before sleeping and put it back on in the morning when she got dressed. The ring was symbolic of the nonmaterial nature that was concealed and revealed to her at times.

She pondered explanations given for the patterns on the butterflies' wings; but ultimately she felt that the beauty of the wings was better realized without thoughts. She wondered why leaves turned colors or rain fell or rainbows appeared after it stormed, and her wonderings led her to a quietude that was fulfilling. It was then that she felt she could see clearly and it was this vision that made her a spiritual teacher. People thought of her as a magician or guardian angel and said she was a seer: watching over them, teaching them how to see. She saw the invisible in the visible and understood what she saw. She worshipped the world: the tree, the butterfly's wings, the grain of rice, and the dust particles . . . without any estrangement.

Sun and Das

On the east side of Manhattan was a school where Clara was first a student and later also a teacher. The school was a place where spiritual teachings and methods were given, as well as the time and space to practice. There was a path that led to the school. The path had been painstakingly built, one step at a time, by two artists, whom it seemed at the time to others and perhaps even to themselves did not know where they were going, yet all along made decisions and acted in ways that revealed they did have a plan after all. The two were called Sun and Das. They were mirrors and the path they built was a path of seeing.

Sun and Das lived in Wooster, a small town on the other side of the mountain, in a brown house tucked in the woods, with two ponds. They grew vegetables, herbs, and flowers. Das grew mugwort and put it in his socks, as it kept the skin on the bottom of his feet soft. He was always working in the garden, had a long beard, and though he didn't say much, was friendly. He wore a knitted hat even on the hottest of summer days. Sun and Das had a lot of knowledge about gardening, and if you wanted to know when to cut back roses or how far under the ground to plant flower bulbs they could tell you. Many people had lost this knowledge and used chemicals to make plants grow, and over time the chemicals destroyed the land.

Clara's garden for the most part remained in her mind. She did not have the strength to turn the soil. Where she lived, the earth was hard as it was mostly clay. Nevertheless, she dreamed of gardens inspired by the paintings of Claude Monet or Pierre-Auguste Renoir and imagined one day having them.

Theo

Clara lived with a thin, tall, handsome man named Theo. Sometimes while driving, he saw flowers on the roadside or in the gardens of what seemed to be abandoned houses. The houses themselves were deteriorating and looked like dying flowers. He sometimes picked these flowers and brought them home. Clara liked having flowers in vases on tables inside, even though she felt bad about their displacement. Hence, opposing thoughts existed in her mind. Looking at the flowers reminded Clara of abandoned houses. She remembered one in particular: a large Victorian with a tower on each side, balconies on the second and third floor, many stained-glass windows, and a porch that wrapped all the way around. Although Clara never saw the inside, she could tell that it would have had at least two staircases and probably a third. To Clara, a house with more than one staircase was a more important house somehow. She loved this house and would go out of her way to walk or drive past it. After some years, the house was torn down. In its place went something so ugly and poorly made that she herself felt wounded.

Meryl

When Clara was in the third grade, she had a classmate named Meryl whose father died in the Vietnam War. Clara didn't know exactly what this meant, only that there was a lot of excitement because her father was finally "coming home" in three and then two weeks, but then he didn't come home. After that, Meryl missed a month of school and when she came back the teacher asked Clara to help Meryl catch up on the work she had missed. Clara did not know what death or war was but sensed that something terrible had happened to Meryl and wanted to be of help.

So she organized her notes to the best of her ability, to be able to share what she'd learned with Meryl. In the midst of Meryl's sorrow, her lessons with Clara were different from the other lessons in the school because Clara was trying to cheer her up, and Clara, unlike many of the other students and even some of the teachers, wasn't afraid of Meryl's grief and didn't try to avoid her. Clara remained a source of learning for Meryl throughout their lives and Meryl thought early on that what they were studying was something larger and more lasting than it appeared.

Before this experience with Meryl, Clara hadn't felt that what she'd been learning in school was all that valuable. But as she passed what she'd learned from her teacher to Meryl, she herself understood the lessons better and developed a deeper appreciation for study. More than that, however, was her sense of responsibility toward Meryl, such that she cared more for Meryl's test results and grades than for her own. These are the types of lessons that are taught in schools only indirectly. These lessons— responsibility, empathy, friendship, camaraderie—are there to be learned all the time, regardless of what day it is, and can flow through and unify all the subjects, whether history, mathematics, English, or gym; subjects we like or not.

Later, when Clara was in high school, the appreciation for learning she'd acquired on Meryl's behalf diminished. No longer feeling Meryl's profound sadness, and no longer being responsible for someone whose father had died in Vietnam, Clara lost interest in her studies and went to school only to meet with friends and then leave, spending much of the day as a delinquent.

Emmet

Clara had a friend named Emmet who also lived on the other side of the mountain, the same side as Sun and Das, on River Road. River Road is one of the most beautiful roads in that area. The houses on River Road are mostly stone houses built in the 1800s and are far apart from each other, separated by stone walls and stone bridges and close enough to the road that one can see them easily. Emmet was a painter and for decades he made watercolors of objects and people that he loved, using the sun, moon, or a candle as his source for light. He had a vision that belonged to an earlier century, where life was slower, bluer, prettier, sadder, and had more pathos and time for drinking tea and arranging plates of fruit. He liked watercolor paint because it was wet and hard to control. He liked the way colors bled into one another, making edges soft and blurry. When Emmet was in his forties, he fell off a ladder and hit his head hard against the floor. Ironically, afterwards, much of what he did see was soft and blurry, but within several months of his fall he completely lost his eyesight. At the time of his fall, something was troubling him, though what it was he kept silent about. Blind, and with his house so close to the road, he would walk into the road and nearly get killed, daily.

Though Emmet could no longer see with his physical eyes, he could see in his mind. He remembered what everything looked like and could describe a painting that he loved better and with more detail than those with sight. He had always loved and collected antiques. When he lost his sight he still continued to build his collection. He lived in one of the oldest houses in Wooster. Everything in his house seemed to belong, and had been perfectly placed in relation to the age and feel of the house. When he was blind, this perfect placement he'd always had became a part of his blindness, in that he knew exactly where everything was because of the importance he assigned to where he had put things. He saw them in his mind, and how he saw them in his mind was how they were. When he could no longer physically see the objects he owned, he loved them no less and kept everything. The line between his physical and mental space was a soft one and he took good care of them both.

Eventually, Emmet found it difficult to be alone as much as he was, so Clara spent more time with him and arranged to be with him on days when he had doctors' appointments or needed provisions so that she could help him walk down the streets of the small but often bustling town of Wooster, where pedestrians stop suddenly to send text messages without considering that someone who may be blind or seeing-impaired is walking behind them. He would put his hand on Clara's shoulder and she guided him. She felt his large hand on her shoulder and felt especially purposeful. Emmet was tall and though blind he wore two pairs of square black eyeglasses, one on top of the other. He was a sharp dresser and Clara always dressed up for him. Clara only wore glasses for reading and though her reading glasses helped her to see words, nothing helped her see her world more clearly than walking with Emmet.

Sometimes Clara made drawings of the flowers that Theo had picked for her. Emmet would ask her to describe her drawings, for he cared and wanted to know. Clara loved these conversations they had together. She wished that he might someday in the future see again. She would often want to "show" something to him. He took his blindness relatively well but the depth of his darkness and loneliness was undeniable as well as his wish to someday see Clara, whom he had never actually seen, and this pained him at times.

Theo

Theo was a great reader and turned to books for wisdom. It was one of his practices. He read with discipline, uninterrupted, for long periods of time and became a better person because of it. He was different from most people around him in many ways—one being that he did not possess a computer or cell phone. He stayed at home reading and borrowed books from the library. They liked him at the library and if they didn't have a book he wanted they would call to have it sent from another library, even if it were far away. Clara tended to read scriptures or religious books, or books about the lives of saints; Theo read fiction, novels, and poetry. He read books about women with powers who understood the seasons and weather; or who had tragic backgrounds and were melancholy and made things up in order to get attention; or who were poor or orphaned, or undergoing an unwanted pregnancy. He read books about men who went to war, committed crimes, or fell in love with women of a different class during an era when it would never have been allowed. He read books about survivors—those who had hidden in basements, escaped through under-ground tunnels; went hungry; knew sacrifice, loyalty, humility, service; and made good out of their lives despite the odds being against them. He read books about children, horses, mothers, death, meal times, bed times, houses in the country with open or closed windows, or empty houses where people had once lived in stormy places where there was lots of wind and no trees for protection. Theo was always reading—early morning, late at night, and in the afternoon. He would often tell Clara about what he was reading and sometimes she would become so interested that she would start reading the book herself. Mostly, however, she enjoyed his versions better.

Theo was a nurse. Where Theo and Clara lived, in the countryside, male nurses were less common than in the city. Theo experienced every-thing as a nurse: amputated limbs, weak hearts, respiratory problems, liver transplants, questions like, "You mean she's not coming home?" or "When can I leave?" or statements like, "I just want to feel good again." He saw death, disease, despair, and deterioration and, alongside, usually some kind of underlying sweetness or pathos, something that touched him and brought out his compassionate side. He was steady in his work, appreci-ated by his coworkers, and not motivated by money, of which he did not make much, or so Clara thought, considering how hard he worked and how close to or at the end many of his patients were. Theo's work made him patient and wise. He had great depth and maturity and perhaps this was why naturally he was not much of a consumer; he wasn't thirsty for what it seems many people are thirsty for. It seems everyone wants something, but Theo didn't have that. He took care of sick people without wanting reward.

Eli

On account of Theo's work and his good disposition, Clara's father, Eli, was pleased with their marriage and they had his blessing. Eli was similar to Theo in that he worked hard, loved his wife, Clara, and rarely bought anything for himself. Eli didn't read novels or poetry, though—perhaps because his own life had been so full of extremes, dramas, and tragedies that he wanted to forget, though he never could. He was a scientist, a good father, a loving husband, and at heart a gentle man, though he was temperamental and sometimes could throw a fit that was alarming. In other words, you didn't want to upset him. Clara upset him at her wedding because he didn't like having his picture taken so many times. She upset him when she was a teenager because she got into trouble frequently. She upset him when she went traveling for several years and only phoned home when she needed money. But most of all she upset him because she didn't have any children.

Clara had a brother named Solon, who had two sons. This meant that Eli did have grandchildren, even if the children didn't belong to Clara. Solon was a doctor and a very religious man who cared greatly for the books and customs of his religion and followed many traditional rules that affected how he dressed, ate, and which days he rested; when he could or could not turn lights on, drive a car, or answer the phone, etc. He knew ancient languages as well as modern medicine, and what had originally seemed dogmatic (at least to Clara) about her brother turned out to be a life full of joy and equipoise. His children were reared reading holy books and hearing stories with morals. They stayed away from television and possessed an innocence about them that, to this day and now grown men (one an astronaut and the other a veterinarian), still remains. Clara was amazed by all of Solon's accomplishments.

Clara liked Solon's wife, Esther, who was born in Japan and grew up with the tradition, culture, and rituals from that part of the world. Though she had lived in America since her teenage years, Esther had ways of doing things so that even how she folded a napkin traced her back to her country. She was practical and present and dreamed of her childhood and upbringing in that distant land. Clara thought of her as exceedingly kind. Like Solon, she was a doctor, but she worked with people who had no money, had slipped through the cracks, were by themselves, and cared for by no one; they were unloved, abandoned, homeless, cold, hungry, soiled, and acutely sick.

Esther loved her work. Whereas Solon enjoyed a great amount of acknowledgment as a doctor, traveled, published articles, and was written about, Esther cared nothing of such things for herself. They had a great love for each other and never fought, which Clara attributed to their religion and to all the rules they followed. It was a way of following patterns that were created so that one felt close to "HaShem," and it seemed to be working for them, especially in their marriage. Eli was skeptical of religion and of such laws and restrictions in general, as he had seen, sadly enough, murder, genocide, holocausts, wars, and hatred connected to people's narrow and misunderstood interpretations of religion. But he had grown over time, as he had to, to accept it in his son.

Eli was a hard worker. He worked so hard that at the end of his life he literally couldn't work anymore, because every time he tried to he'd fall asleep. His life of war, sickness, struggle, love, and the worry that went with that love, and his temperament—gentle, yet volatile all the same— exhausted him. He had an enlarged heart, swollen ankles, and a rounded back such that his shoulders were higher than his ears. He had large brown eyes, distinguished lips, wrinkles, and gray hair that he had even before Clara had been born. When Clara was a child most of her friends thought Eli was her grandfather, and Clara thought most of her friend's fathers seemed more like brothers, someone to play basketball with but not old enough to be a father. Eli was old at forty and lived to be ninety-two. Clara had wished Eli could have lived longer, but once he became incontinent, he no longer wanted to live.

Sarah

Eli was married to Sarah, Clara and Solon's mother. Sarah could have been an extraordinary actress and loved the theater. She was also a talented painter and writer, and probably could have been a successful artist. Instead, she was a dedicated, loving, patient, and thoughtful wife, mother, and housekeeper. She did act, paint, and write but didn't pursue it with the rigor that she might have, had she not put her family first. She was naturally a creative person; she learned languages quickly, understood accents of class and geography, and could voice these accents perfectly, with ease and fluidity. She was an incredible storyteller and could talk about nothing and/or everything in ways that people loved. She had a rich life to draw from, like Eli, with a background of war and many stories of loss and survival in her head.

Sarah, like Theo, was also not an excessive consumer. She attributed this to growing up wealthy, in a household full of servants, tailors, cooks, and maids, where three generations of her family lived together in a grandly ornate building, from the Art Deco period, in the best part of Berlin, Germany. Sarah had two nannies all to herself, as she said, "One to braid the right side, and one to braid the left side," of her hair. The family ate sixteen-course meals, in a room full of paintings by Max Beckmann and Ernst Ludwig Kirchner; the cutlery was pure silver and the frames around the paintings were gold. Sarah's parents had annual box seats at the opera and her mother had a reputation for being the best-dressed woman in town. Sarah remembers as a child her mother entering her bedroom to say *goodnight* on her way to the opera or some such cultural event, dressed in a sequined gown and wearing long, diamond earrings.

All of that came to an abrupt end with the war, which left Sarah's family with nothing but the clothes on their backs, quite literally, and a diet of nothing but potatoes, cooked in a land that she had escaped to but could never call home. This harsh experience had left her completely unattached and without any sentiment toward things. She turned away from the label of *refugee* and the regret of lost wealth, and embraced family life, just as Clara's father had turned away from his bitterness over having to leave behind his home and birthplace due to the war, and embraced science.

The lives of Clara's parents were geared toward family, the arts, and sciences. Neither Clara nor Solon were spoiled, and were not given things as children as incentives to behave well if they were good. Perhaps because of these influences, Clara had a certain amount of determination to make something out of her life.

The Abbot

Near to where Clara lived, at the top of Pine Forest Mountain, was a Tibetan monastery. Clara had been curious about it for years. She knew that nuns and monks were in residence there, as well as an abbot in seclusion who was almost ninety years old and highly respected. She had heard that for the weekend of his ninetieth birthday he would come out of seclusion to give teachings and tell stories of the Buddha. These teachings would be given in Tibetan and then translated, as the abbot did not speak English. When Clara heard which weekend it was, she planned on going, and Theo wanted to accompany her. This was swell because she enjoyed being with Theo and she was afraid of the drive up the mountain, which was steep and unfamiliar.

Theo made the drive in half the amount of time it would have taken Clara, past old houses and rose bushes to an area where houses were beginning to be spread further apart from each other the higher up the mountain they drove. At the highest point, like churches in Europe often are, with grand views of below, was the monastery. It looked like monasteries Clara had seen in India, and with the weather being rainy and the sky overcast, she thought of times in her past where she'd visited similar places in similar weather, in what was called the monsoon or rainy season. Clara liked the monsoon. Too many bright days in a row she found difficult.

Theo and Clara followed the walking path from the road to the main gate. Inside the main gate was an overgrown garden, where weeds seemed appreciated and were left to flower as they pleased. This pleased Clara: the wildness of the land. Theo and Clara took their shoes off and went inside the temple.

Once, many years back when Clara was in India, she was not allowed inside a particular temple because it was only for men. So at five AM in the morning, having gone early to hear the low voices of the monks in prayer, she sat outside the doors, which were open, so she could see inside and thereby still feel a part of it. At various times, the monks from inside brought her tea, bread, and a mat to sit on, and asked her where she was from. Some of the nuns, who also weren't allowed inside, came and joined her. Clara was happy they joined her, as they made her feel that she belonged.

Back at the monastery on top of the mountain, only a few nuns were inside, meditating. Theo and Clara were early. When Clara walked in, she faced the golden Buddha. All around the Buddha were paintings depicting the story of his enlightenment. Altars stood in front, to the left and to the right of the Buddha, with glasses of fresh water and candles burning on top. The altars were tended to differently than the outdoor gardens. The objects of worship on the altars were placed according to instructions found in scriptures that contained diagrams and nothing was left to chance.

The glasses were well organized: in rows, with exactly the same amount of water in each glass, and each glass the same distance apart from another. The candles were precisely placed on beautiful cloths. Vases of flowers and bells used for ringing at different times during the worship were arranged with great care. Nothing was random. Clara was excited once inside. She loved the atmosphere and had in fact at one time in her life fantasized about being a nun. Her husband had even said that if she were to ever leave him (which she knew she never would), it would be for the nunnery and not another man.

Clara noticed prayer sheets on the table at the far left of the room and went to see what they were, while Theo moved directly to his seat. Clara found various sets of prayers: those of offerings, dedications, supplications, and lists of the bodhisattva vows and the various lineages. She took one of each set of prayers, in her usual way of wanting to learn, and went and sat by Theo. She began reading the prayers, for there was an English translation provided under the Tibetan script. The prayers described visions, flowers, clouds, colors, and sounds, all in praise of the Buddha. She loved reading these prayers and had spread the sheets around her on the floor when a monk appeared, took all the papers, lifted them off the floor, and slid a wooden platform underneath them. He smiled at Clara, and she understood immediately that such sheets did not belong on the floor. In fact, she knew that already, but at that moment, when she was reading, she'd in some way forgotten the etiquette around their sacredness and was happy to be reminded of this by the monk.

Time passed: the abbot arrived and the sets of prayers were sung. They were long and when everyone completed singing them, the abbot said in Tibetan, which his student translated, "Now we will begin again," and everyone started once more. The prayers were sung three times. Clara tried her best to keep up. She did not understand Tibetan but felt mysteriously like she knew the language and the whole setting was familiar to her.

At the time when Clara was singing these prayers, she was fifty-three years old. When she was twenty, she had broken many bones in her body. So now, as an older woman, though she was graceful in her body and enjoyed various forms of movement and dance, her back tired easily and she had a habit of slouching. She thought that even without having broken so many bones, she probably would still slouch on account of having watched her father do the same, progressively worse each year, until his back was so curved it was painful simply to look at him. Eli suffered a lot of pain and this was evident just by the slow way that he sat down and even slower way he got back up.

So, Clara, trying hard to read the prayers now placed on the platform but still quite a distance from her middle-aged eyes, was slouching when the same monk from before appeared, picked up the prayer sheets, and slid another platform on top of the platform already there. Then he raised a little bookstand that was built into the platform for the papers to lean against, so that now Clara could straighten her back and look directly at the papers. She thanked the monk, who smiled at her, and felt that God had touched her through the care that the monk had shown, not only for the prayers but also for her wellbeing.

It was experiences like this, which Clara had often, that gave her a feeling of recovery. More and more such experiences were happening to her and in their progression she believed that this feeling of recovery, if felt by others, would awaken the natural inclination in others to want to save the forests and trees from being cut down. She understood that if the trees were not enough in number, the mud underneath her feet and the feet of those around her and far from her, would slide. Thus, she felt the stability of the land and of her life tied together. She often thought that the chopping down of a tree was like cutting oneself off from one's natural evolution, like cutting one's potential or wisdom in half.

The abbot celebrated his ninetieth birthday and after the morning session he retired to his room and the nuns and monks stayed and discussed what a great master he was, and how all of his wishes over the years had come true. It was said that his wishes were never motivated by personal gain—never, not even once—and that whenever there had been problems at the monastery the abbot never turned toward the material world to solve them. People said that the abbot felt close to the Buddha, much closer to the Buddha than to the things around him, like his clothes or the table or the pot of tea. In the monastery and all that she encountered there, Clara saw a reality that deeply stirred her.

Frances

Theo's mother Frances was ninety-one. She had a lot in common with Eli and Sarah in that she was also a survivor: she had lived through war, poverty, hunger, tuberculosis, and despair. From the age of five, she had been asking "Why?" about everything. Inquiring was what she lived for and it kept her going. She lived in an apartment on Eighteenth Street in New York City. She had lived there since leaving the suburbs of New Jersey, which she hated, after her husband's sudden death from a heart attack that Theo thought was caused by the fact that his father was a salesman when in reality he didn't believe in selling things. At that time, Frances was forty-five, had two teenage children, and had been married sixteen years. She never remarried, because in her mind, in some way, she was still married even though her husband was no longer alive.

The death of Frances's husband weighed heavily on her and her children. However, as time passed it caused her to become much more independent than she thought would have happened had he lived. Her apartment was in the back of a building with eight floors. It had at one time been a dentist's office. This made sense with relation to the layout of the apartment, which had small rooms off a long and narrow hallway. It was quiet and overlooked a completely uncared-for garden that was encroached upon by the never-ending construction around it, which was taking place all around the world as well: an obsession with buildings and concrete. At her age, Frances no longer knew any of the people who lived in the building, which itself was not well looked-after since the owner (a hard-working immigrant from Greece) had died and his son, born in America and not hard-working at all, had inherited the building.

The back room of Frances's apartment, which faced the garden, extended further than the rest of the building, so there was nothing built on top of it. The roof of that room was in serious need of repair; any time it rained, water leaked in. Years went by with water dripping in, and the landlord always said he'd send somebody over to have a look or fix it. But no one ever came. Or someone came but the landlord was never willing to pay anyone properly, so even a good workman couldn't fix the roof because they weren't given the amount of money it would take to do so.

At the age of ninety-one, Frances, who'd once liked rain, unfortunately had grown to dislike it because it meant she'd be on her hands and knees wiping the floor dry with towels, collecting water in buckets, and then, when those buckets got too heavy, going out into the street and looking for someone she assessed as decent to come in and help her lift the buckets and empty them out. This habit of hers of leaving the apartment to look for someone to invite inside to move heavy things concerned her son, but Frances had her own way of doing things.

Clara had a wonderful relationship with Frances and it was agreed that she would look upon Frances not as a mother-in-law but as a second mother. She would visit Frances on Sundays, when she came to the city to teach. One Sunday, Frances wanted to talk about *Anna Karenina*, as she'd just finished reading it. She read with glasses but they were glasses she'd purchased for a few dollars at the drugstore and they magnified things only slightly. Clara and Theo both thought it was unusual and inspiring that Frances, at age ninety-one, could still read long books with small print with these simple glasses.

So, Frances in her relatively dark, ground-floor apartment, having outlived almost everyone and not one to go out anymore unless she needed help emptying a full bucket of rainwater or opening or closing a heavy window, was having deep and original thoughts about Tolstoy's novel. According to Frances, Anna's story was a cover for the real story, which had to do with Levin. Levin was a member of the aristocracy but he fell in love with and married a peasant. Because of his connections to the aristocracy, he tried to help the peasant family of his wife (Frances couldn't remember her name, which was Katerina, or Kitty) and improve the situation in general of the peasants whose lives were lived in stark contrast to those of the aristocracy. Frances identified strongly with the peasants and with those who wanted to expose injustice.

In this way, through her reading, Frances was brought to a place inside herself where questions and answers turned into understanding and truth. She found her reading and the discussions she had with her children about her reading meaningful and a main source of a higher level of satisfaction that other things could not provide. She thought that Clara should read *Anna Karenina*, especially the last fifty pages, and tried to get her to read them then and there, on that specific occasion. "Just read it now," she kept saying. But Clara did not have time nor was she in the right mindset, and she was happy merely to communicate with someone who'd just read Tolstoy.

Whatever it was that Clara and Frances discussed—whether it was the weather: rain, freezing rain, flurries, or snow; whether it was their moods, health, or the food they'd been eating—they helped each other to contemplate and reflect on their lives and life in general, and in this way their visits were meaningful. They appreciated one another and what the other had to say. Clara always left Frances feeling happy and Frances shared in that same expansive feeling when Clara left.

Clara knew that Frances would not live forever, in the way she had thought her father would. Eli had died, and there were others, too—some old, but others not; some expected to die, and others not—and Clara realized that loved ones could pass at any moment. She could see that Frances's body, like Sarah's, and even her own, was deteriorating and impermanent. She could see that it was slipping away, but knew that the impression that Frances had made on her would go on, even when Frances was no longer in her physical form. Clara thought Frances's influence would always support her even if Frances no longer had the support of her body. Clara imagined a time in the future where it would no longer be necessary to enjoy or delight in Frances's form. She imagined that at that time she would know Frances to be the blue sky.

Frances also knew she was dying. She had a routine of exercises, which included walking to the front and back of the apartment five times or sitting down in a chair, standing up, sitting back down, and standing back up fifteen times. She questioned the point of these exercises, encouraged to do them by her children. Since she was no longer as active as she had once been, she often felt each day physically less capable than the day before. But then she'd go through periods where she did see some improvement (she assumed on account of her exercises), and she described this as "turning around."

Unlike her body, her mind was not deteriorating. She forgot words and where she put things, but she could concentrate on a piece of music, meditate on the beauty of a flower, pause and rest in the depth of silence, and was skillful in her relationships with her children. She was willing to let go of her grip on her body and the externals around it. She had faith in God, whom she referred to as a great mystery, one whose meaning would only be diminished through words. She had the stamina to keep her surroundings (her clothes, refrigerator, and bathtub) clean without any help, which she always refused when either of her children offered. Her long-term memory was sharp. She remembered starving as a child, passages from Dante and Homer, Italian and Latin grammar, European history, and all the specialty shops in New York City: one for bread, one for thread, one for olive oil, etc. that she used to go to. Most of those stores were no longer there or had moved to where she could no longer find them.

She remembered the clothes she made by hand for her children and how her children didn't like them. She remembered that she used to walk ninety blocks and then cook for five people and then go to a movie. She remembered various schoolteachers: kind ones she loved, mean ones she feared; and often being told by authority figures as a child not to ask so many questions. Most important about Frances, at least to Clara, was that Frances was preoccupied with the wellbeing and happiness of others. She worried about war and poverty and people being exploited whom she did not know, who were far away yet part of her concern. Though she rarely left her apartment, she was not closed off.

Having come from Italy, Frances worked for eight years in New York City as a teacher of Italian after her husband died. In the school where she worked was a man from Morocco who was teaching French. Work was rarely offered to him; he was the last one on the list to be called. Frances thought the reason for this was that he was poorly dressed, his clothes were torn or dirty, and he was shabby-looking and smelled bad. She sometimes thought she should tell him that if he wanted more work he should improve his appearance, but she could never tell him this because she thought it would humiliate him. She also sensed that he was poor and hungry; so instead of telling him about his clothes, she brought him plates of spaghetti. Years later, she still thought about this man.

Sun and Das

Clara met Sun and Das when she was in her early twenties. At that time, they, like her, lived in New York City. They both had long hair. Sun had a green streak in hers, wore a purple velvet cloak, and played the violin. They had a mildness about them, in that if you had to have a medical procedure it would be good to hold on to one of their hands. It would be calming. They looked more at ease than most people and didn't seem so strained. At the same time, there was an intensity about them. They wanted to make a difference, a change, to be part of an awakening that mainly focused on getting people to stop eating animals. They did not feel they could rest while thousands of animals were being slaughtered daily. They lived on vegetables and grains and were the picture of health. They never aged and continued to grow more and more attractive.

Clara also did not eat animals. This began for her when she was thirteen. Eli had taken her for a sandwich and the piece of meat that she was eating was tough and difficult to chew. She asked her father what it was she was actually eating. Throughout her childhood, her family had spent two weeks out of every year in the Adirondack Mountains. These were her favorite two weeks of the year because Eli was around the whole time; the rest of the year, he was always working. During these two weeks, uniquely, he wore a lightweight plaid jacket. In the area where the family stayed were many farms. Cows were grazing on the land, and Eli was always taking Clara to see them.

Seeing the cows was part of their vacation. When Clara couldn't chew her piece of meat, her father explained that it was the flesh of the cows he had shown her when they were vacationing and he was wearing his plaid jacket. She felt ashamed and decided never again to eat meat . . . animals. So when Sun and Das and Clara first met each other, they had something that was important to them in common. Clara felt instantly that she could spend the rest of her life with Sun and Das. So when Sun told her she should go to India, that an enlightened teacher with spiritual wisdom lived there, she went. Three days later.

Wise One

Clara saw kindness and love personified in this enlightened teacher. Everyone called him simply "teacher" or "Wise One." In Clara's eyes, he was perfect. Clara had a small box where she kept her money. She wanted to give all the money that was in this small box to him. She wanted to approach Wise One and offer him her life. Wise One sent her to the nearby village where she helped his friends Rupa and Vidya, who had a clinic for children and young adults who were called "slow" by society but thought of as special by the friends of Wise One.

Rupa and Vidya were not a couple in the usual sense. They lived together in the same guesthouse, which belonged to the clinic, but they weren't married or romantic with one another in the way that Clara and Theo were. They each had their own bedroom and everything else they shared. Years ago, they had turned the earth and built the clinic with their own hands. They loved children and wanted to give those who needed special attention a chance to work at a slower pace, and to provide an education. This education included painting, learning English, making chocolates, gardening, crafting rugs, and baking bread, among other things. When the children graduated they had enough skills to earn at least a little money, enough so their families wouldn't turn them out on the street.

The children were very gifted and Clara bought many paintings and chocolates from them. She spent most of her time there giving love and affection to the children. She found she had a lot of love to give. Later on in her life, when she looked back on that time at the clinic, she felt it was one of the happiest because in some small way she felt useful: to the children and, indirectly, to Wise One. This "work" that Clara did with the children was the beginning of her forgetting her nervousness and anxiety. Her focus was on the children and not on herself. This was a great relief and one of the first important teachings she received from Wise One.

When Clara arrived in India it was hot, muggy, and the air was thick. She took a bus from the airport to the bus station. The bus drove through a slum behind the airport, which was unlike anything she had seen before. When she got to the bus station it was the middle of the night and she had to wait several hours for the first bus of the day to take her to where she was going. The bus station was a little scary at that hour but a tea stall was open, so she went in. The man who was making the tea seemed good-natured and she decided to spend the next few hours in the safety of the tea stall and in the course of the night drank many cups; the tea was extra sweet and she liked it.

When she arrived in the town of Sarana, where the enlightened teacher lived, she had already seen enough of India to know that it was different from America, yet she felt at home. Already she desired to purchase a sari and dress like the Indian women. She checked into a small, modest, but clean hotel that Sun and Das had told her about. She rested, bathed, and then followed a map hand-drawn by Das to the enlightened teacher's house. When the house was in sight, Clara saw an older man peeking out of the door, such that one foot was inside the house and the other on the landing. He looked straight at her as if he was expecting her, as if she was a daughter or a relation whom he had been hoping and waiting for. He was smiling, laughing, and waving his hand, telling her, "You come. You come." She picked up her pace, which was rare for her, and before long she was inside the house.

Wise One accepted Clara as his student. He taught her how to move and breathe in a way that would change her forever. He had learned these systems and principles from his teacher. He made a point of stressing that he'd invented nothing in his teaching; all of it had come from his teacher. When Wise One spoke of his teacher he would start crying. Wise One was a special soul, untouched and not entangled by personal drama. He was free from his own afflictions and existed for the sake of guiding others. Clara found in this relationship shelter, safety, and rest. She felt in his presence, and even not in his presence but just through his association or blessing, that no harm could come to her. From this refuge, so full of affection and trust, Clara's ability to learn increased and Wise One shared his knowledge with her.

Each day that she came to class, when the house was just in sight, he'd be standing in the doorway, one foot in the house and one on the landing, waving, telling, "You come. You come." She loved being in his house and felt his family members to be extensions of him, such that many years later, when Wise One left his body, she felt almost the same way being with his daughter Mira or grandson Hari as she did with him.

* * *

Years later, when Clara was still travelling to India, even after Wise One was no longer in his body, Clara continued to visit and work for Rupa and Vidya, who needed more help than before because their hard work had aged them.

One evening after a long day of study and work, Clara went for a walk. It was the time of day when day was ending but still not completely over, and night was just about to begin, and the line between day and night was slow and soft. Indian people like to be out at that time. The light was beautiful, more pink than yellow. Sarana was too big to be a village but too small and village-like to be a town. It was traditional in many ways: women still wore saris, men still wore dhotis and wrapped towels around their heads, and most people ate with their right hand. Families sat on the front stoops of their houses, which were small and attached to one another, with the front doors open so that one could see inside. The women were occupied with some form of housework, the children were doing their homework, the men were enjoying a smoke, and the elderly were watching as life passed them by.

While Clara was walking she heard many sounds: but one sound, that of singing, enchanted her and she stood still and listened. Then, without thinking, she followed the sound of the music to where it was coming from. The music came from a particular house, and as she walked up to it she saw many sets of shoes and sandals lined up on the porch and knew that the shoes must belong to the singers. She let herself into the house. The music was coming from the second floor and she climbed the stairs. At the top, just off the landing, was a small corner room with windows on two sides, such that the light of day was even lovelier inside than out. Thirty men, women, and children were sitting cross-legged on the floor, men on one side, women on the other. It was hard to believe that thirty people could fit into such a tiny room, but Indians are used to and seem to like sitting close to each other.

They all faced a large picture of a man whom Clara recognized as Sri Sathya Sai Baba, a highly respected and popular saint, part of a line of incarnations of great saints of India. Though it was only a picture and Sai Baba was no longer in his body, the people were singing to the picture as if their beloved was in their presence in that room, and Clara felt it, too. The mood of devotion: the flowers, the smells, the music, the tonality—slightly dissonant even painful; haunting, yet melodious; the lack of anything artificial, mechanical, pretentious—pulled her inside. The women moved over for her, and Clara, tall compared to the others in the room, took her seat, feeling as if in a boat on a journey, going somewhere that would always be new and praiseworthy. She was happy in this room. She felt connected to the sounds, the people, and the tiny, crowded space. She felt that she belonged. She felt included. She thought of her shoes on the porch as part of the group of old and worn shoes.

These thoughts relaxed her and she joined in and began singing. One of the ladies brought her a sheet where the songs were written in English so that she could sing along. When it was over everyone filed out. At the bottom of the stairs an elderly man spooned a few drops of rosewater and saffron-infused liquid into each person's cupped hands. Clara watched each person receive the liquid, take a sip, and then place the rest on the top of his or her head. She thought it was graceful, like a dance, and that these external customs created a sacred atmosphere while something internal was happening, so that as she felt drawn out toward the others and all that the night entailed, she also felt pulled inward, so that inside of that house she found her Self.

Clara

Clara loved to sing and lived in a world of song and musicality. She liked to sing scales and simple sounds over and over again. She also sung from old philosophical texts that were poetic and abstract. She learned things through singing that she felt she could not have learned in other ways. Singing helped her to feel stable and in her stability discover what she had forgotten. Sometimes, while singing, she would become elevated and at the peak of her concentration think of some chore needing to be done. She would negotiate with herself whether to stop singing or not. Mostly, she let those thoughts pass, continued her singing, and allowed herself to go deep into her reverie. Gradually, these thoughts of chores disappeared completely and she became absorbed in and captivated by her song. Eventually, she sang while doing chores, and the chore inspired further songs, so that they were no longer chores in a mundane sense.

* * *

When Clara finished high school, she had no desire to go to college, even though her father and mother both thought it would be best. When Clara, at the age of fifty, looked back on her life, reflecting on who she'd been as a young adult, it was "as if" (for Clara in her adult studies of philosophy had thought many times over the words *as if*) she'd been another person. She had misconstrued a lot of false ideas about herself and others, and was distracted, restless, unkind, and selfish. She told lies about many things all the time and couldn't remember what she'd told to whom. She couldn't keep her stories straight and in her own mind lost track of what had "really happened." She sniffed powders and smoked weeds and swallowed tablets, and while under the influence of psychedelics saw imaginary colors in the ether when she waved her hands. She did these things often, and hated that she did, but continued doing them anyway. But all of that stopped when she had a car accident and broke many bones and was left nearly paralyzed. She lay in bed for months, unable to move. Her pain was so great that she was not in pain; she was removed from it, above or to the side of it; an onlooker, spared somehow. Then one day, she lifted a finger and moved a toe and gradually got her feeling back. After that time, she relinquished her unkindness and distraction. Her attitude completely changed. She became nicer and more caring. Several years later, she met Sun and Das, who blessed her by their kindness and wisdom.

Moses

Clara had a friend named Moses who was like a brother to her. She saw a lot of her own qualities in Moses and he endeared himself to her. Moses had experienced a family tragedy when he was twelve and this left him, for a time, unsure of things, especially himself. Even though he had many great qualities, a circle of friends, and a beautiful loving wife, and had learned many lessons, he yearned for acknowledgment. He tried hard to live a good life and not let his poor habits take over, but often he felt like something was not quite right; that something was missing, wrong, or off. Because of that, he was often worried and couldn't settle down. On really tough days he felt disconnected from others, God, and himself. Most of the time, this unanchored feeling was slight, but occasionally it took over.

One day when he was feeling dismal, he went for a walk. He came upon a field of grass, turned, and walked into the field. Not knowing why, he took off his shoes. He had not been barefoot outside in a long time. The grass felt wet and cold and this felt good to him. He put his bag down. He was always carrying unnecessary items, as this was symptomatic of his insecurity. Carrying things made him feel more secure, but at the same time weighed him down. He was sometimes unintentionally careless, and would say things he didn't mean. He would spend his time watching television even when there wasn't anything worth watching and this always made him feel bad because he knew that life was precious. Sometimes he would have an appetite for something; he would give it to himself, even though he actually had no real desire or affection for it.

Like many people who experience tragedy, Moses turned to God. He kept an altar with pictures of sages and family members, including the family member whose outcome had been so heartbreaking. He sat quietly every morning before this altar. He lit candles and cried. He prayed for a pure vision, not a wrong or mistaken one. He loved his wife, Madeleine, and his two cats (one of whom also unexpectedly and tragically died, without any time for preparation). Through prayer and meditation, Moses was able to establish equilibrium, but he could not maintain this feeling of wholeness, which he longed for. It would come but then it would go. Sometimes his struggle was such that he could not even bring himself to sit before his altar. For this he felt regret and then that regret prevented him from sitting before his altar, so he would get into these downward cycles where he turned away from what the altar provided. When he turned away it was painful, not only for him but also for Madeleine. She wondered when he would recover.

So, when Moses, having gone for a walk and having put his unnecessary bags down, and having taken off his shoes and socks, stood barefoot in a field of grass, this small excursion gave him a feeling of serenity and he sat down. He was wearing light-colored pants and the thought of the pants getting dirty occurred to him. But in the spirit of the field of grass and the vision of wild flowers, he let that worry go. He noticed a lunar moth. It had spots on it and antennae. Moses looked closely at the insect and was struck by its beauty. The insect was walking up a blade of grass. He thought that the insect, when it reached the top of that blade, would want to move to the next nearest blade. So, watching the insect carefully, more carefully than he'd watched anything in a long time, he pushed with his finger the next nearest blade of grass toward the moth when it reached the top, and the insect climbed across. Having made things easier for the insect delighted him. He decided to lie down.

Moses looked up at the sky. The sky was open and vast, and though entirely different from the insect, in point of view it seemed to him at that moment that the insect was part of the sky, the sky a part of the insect, he a part of the sky and insect, and the sky and insect part of him. This feeling of exchange and communion he had felt before, but not in a while. It, therefore, felt newfound and he was happy.

Moses got up to walk home, looked down at his socks and shoes, and felt blessed to have them. As he put them on, he thanked his feet for all the walking they do for him. He picked up his bags and vowed to stop carrying so much; it only made him feel inadequate to have to cling to things. He envisioned switching to a small shoulder bag.

When he got home, workmen were in the kitchen. He had forgotten that he and Madeleine had bought a new refrigerator; he was meant to have been there to help with the installation and Madeleine had been wondering where he'd been. The kitchen seemed out of order and the work that the men were doing was noisy. He wanted to leave the apartment and go back to the field of grass: to the flowers, butterflies, insects, and blue sky. She started telling him who had called, who had sent electronic mail. She mentioned that the new refrigerator was not exactly what they'd ordered or expected, that maybe it was too big.

Moses started to feel his newfound feeling slipping away, impinged upon, being taken from him. He felt some resentment, enough to begin again once more his downward cycle. He remembered his family tragedy and as he thought about the whys and what ifs and all the things around the story and his life that disturbed him; his mind was troubled. He became restless and jumpy and while he tried, especially after the workmen left, to listen to Madeleine, he was distracted and began to breathe heavily. In that moment, there wasn't anything she could do.

When Moses's spirits were low he was hard to be with in that he was easily irritated and overlooked the goodness around him, even that of Madeleine. She would make suggestions, try to get him to sit before his altar or practice his guitar or write poetry to collect his scattered mind and bring it into focus. She was concerned with removing his sorrow; she understood his negativity—it was something he shared with all of humanity, even if he had a greater portion of it than she did. Her compassion was large and she was the perfect wife for Moses and Moses was the perfect husband for Madeleine. Through his continuous hard work, Moses grew into a secure peaceful and happy man who had all the more depth and compassion on account of his transformation. The obstacles and suffering that he had to go through, he endured, always persisting in his spiritual quest. His ability to connect to others was heightened by his awareness of the human condition. People felt accepted, unjudged, and understood by Moses and could feel the depth of his desire to be of service and live authentically.

Madeleine

Madeleine was a thoughtful person with a lot of integrity who was gracious and discreet. She was beautiful, with long blond hair, deeply set large green eyes, and long eyelashes. Though she wasn't curvaceous, she was still feminine. Sometimes she wore deep purple eye shadow and people couldn't help but stare. Because of her lack of vanity, her beauty was not threatening or off-putting; it never was, as it can sometimes be, a barrier. Instead, it brought out the beauty in others.

Madeleine respected the Earth and Earthlings and wanted to cause the least harm possible to the planet and its inhabitants. She was careful in this regard and lived by precepts that she adhered to strictly. She avoided all things "disposable." She carried a reusable cup to fill with water when she was away from home, and a container, utensils, and cloth napkin for when she got a salad to go. She brought her own bowl to the movies for popcorn to avoid wasting one single paper bag. She gave most of her money away to anybody that needed it more than she did. She adopted cats and took more time and pleasure in feeding them than she did in feeding herself. When she heard of someone else's suffering she cried as if it was her own, and she always found something to do in response that did actually, if not remove, at least share that suffering, such that the suffering would be easier because it was shared.

Madeleine was idealistic and spent her time constructively. She and Moses had a marriage where sorrow, joy, despair, hope, and the positive and negative could coexist because of their love. Their love for each other was inspiring and attracted others. They were both teachers who taught methods for lifting oneself out of sorrow. They opened a school that was at first small because of their humility but through love the school grew quite large. They built a dynamic community of people who were active in protecting the land, its rivers and forests. Many of them were musical and enjoyed singing and writing poetry and found ways of using their skills and talents to serve others. People of all ages, backgrounds, and circumstances felt welcome there. It became a meeting place where friendships were made and people, with the example of Madeleine and Moses, shared in the pleasures and pains of each other and celebrated each other's virtues. Over the many years that the school was in existence the community thrived without the usual jealousies, judgments, and fault-findings that can bring a community down. Those who got to spend time with Moses and Madeleine were incredibly fortunate, and for most it was life changing.

Sun and Das

Sun and Das knew how to grow vegetables. They hadn't always known this because they'd lived in cities for most of their lives. But moving into the forest led them back to the earth. It was as if the earth had been waiting for them and as soon as they planted the first seeds, there was always abundance. Besides cultivating gardens of vegetables and herbs, Sun had a flower garden. In this garden grew primarily roses, of all different colors and sizes. Sun trimmed them back and covered them with burlap and hay over the winters, and each year the bushes grew back fuller. She never cut them for her own sake, to bring flowers inside. She enjoyed them outside, looking at them through her windows, walking past them on her way through the garden, or even sitting by them outside while studying an ancient language, or a text on alchemy, or a biography of someone she esteemed and took an interest in, like a great renaissance painter or sixteenth-century poet. In addition to the vegetable garden and the rose garden were many wild edibles, mushrooms, and weeds, growing behind their house. Das learned through speaking with the elders whose spirits remained in the forest what was safe to eat and what was poisonous.

Inside their house was a long, narrow wooden table that comfortably fitted twelve people, five on each side and one at each end. Above the table hung an old crystal chandelier that had probably at one time had candles as its light source, and later was converted to gas, and then to electricity. The light that it provided was soft and yellow. Sun loved glass and had a collection of glasses from all over the world. These glasses were mostly presented to her as gifts, as it was known that she liked glass. Because of the gardens, table, chandelier, and the general disposition of hospitality and desire to bring others together that came naturally to Sun and Das, there were often dinners at their house. These dinners were made up of combinations of foods from the garden and from the wild and they tasted of the earth, which meant there was a wholesomeness to their flavor that felt like from another time, when vegetables were grown with respect.

There was an old large mirror on one end of the dining room and since the other end presented windows to the outside, if you looked in the mirror you saw the soft yellow light; the chandelier; the glasses from around the world laid out on the table; two candles usually lit, one at each end of the table; and the nature from the outside, which changed according to the weather and season. Anyone having dinner there, or just standing at the far, window end of the room, would look through the mirror. Because of the age of the mirror, its thickness and the imperfections in the glass, it provided a dreamlike quality to the already dreamlike room. One accepted the soft light, the table setting, the view of the outdoors contained in the mirror indoors, and the atmosphere of kindness, as an offering of serenity—a gift, a ritual, an acknowledgment of life's cycles.

Emmet

After Emmet's fall, he made a promise to God that if he should survive he would live a life that would inspire others; whether it would be as an artist, a caretaker, or a teacher, he did not know. As it turned out, whatever he did was inspirational because of his acceptance of his blindness. It was hard to understand how he could accept being blind since he loved and appreciated beauty so much. But he had a sense that his life belonged to a cycle larger than he could comprehend: one that was God-given and included his blindness.

Emmet and Clara frequently made trips to the art museum—she with her eyes open, he with his eyes closed. He would ask, "Where are we?" "Which wing?" "Which room?" "Which century?" and she described to the best of her ability the Japanese scroll, Dutch genre painting, African textile, Iranian plate, early nineteenth-century photograph, or Impressionist watercolor. With each descriptive detail Clara gave, Emmet would have a question that caused her to look deeper into whatever it was she was looking at. She was amazed by the questions he asked her. If the painting had a vase with flowers in it, he would ask, "How many flowers?" so that Clara would have to count the number of flowers in the vase. When she would tell him, "Five flowers," or "Seven" or, "Too many to count" . . . he would say, "Oh, I see," conveying that that number was significant to him. In this way, Clara learned how to see what she was seeing; Emmet taught her how to read art.

Whenever they got together, Emmet would ask Clara what she was wearing and because of this she would get dressed up and make herself look especially pretty. She knew he'd ask to touch her dress; would want to know what color it was, what the fabric was, where it had come from, and whether it was costly. Emmet himself was sensitive to the feel of fabric, and liked cotton—particularly *khadi*, an Indian homespun cotton cloth that was lightweight and airy. He liked shirts that came from India with high collars and side pockets, Gandhi-style. He liked old shirts from France made of linen with puffy sleeves and he looked remarkable in them. Actually, in certain ways, to Clara, Emmet's blindness made him more attractive and maybe he knew this. He inspired her, as he did most everyone he met, because he always felt so blessed. He saw his blindness as part of a grand scheme and accepted it in the way that a farmer accepts that a certain number of his vegetables will be eaten by worms. He rarely complained. In his appreciation for things as seemingly small as fresh air coming in through the window, he was less needy than most people. It was always a relief to be with him, or even for Clara, just to know that he was there.

34

After Eli passed away, Clara became possessive of his objects. But Eli had not had many material objects and while Clara was grieving, Sarah, who was also grieving, sold all of his possessions for next to nothing, so by the time Clara realized that she wanted some objects that had belonged to her father, most of them were already gone. Her father had a lot of button-down shirts, white with blue stripes, with one chest pocket on the left or right side. These pockets held his eyeglasses and one or two pens. Clara sentimentalized that her father's shirts were imbued with his long life, tiredness, and hard work. Whomever Sarah had sold or given them to would not feel these things. They would not see the man who had worn these shirts, loved his family, and was hunched over.

Clara had to accept the loss of Eli's shirts, as Emmet accepted his blindness. Clara was left with photos of Eli she had taken over the many years of his life. She found that looking at these photos of her father at different ages in his striped shirts in different places—inside, in the house; outside, by the lake; when the family was on vacation, in his plaid jacket—helped her in time to relinquish her grip on her father's body. As her sorrow subsided, so did the darkness she had been in, and she found comfort in the one object that she did have: an old tattered gray sweater, the sweater he had once worn. She wore it often.

Arun

Clara had a friend named Arun who was born in India and lived there until he went to college and decided to study abroad. He studied architecture and engineering and since he had grown up under the influence of his father, a well-known astrologer who always considered the stars when making plans of importance, Arun had a great sense of time and space, place, and design. So when Sun and Das wanted to make changes to their school Clara introduced them to Arun so he could advise them best how to expand and make repairs and at the same time sanctify the school further.

Sun and Das wanted to add several windows high up so there would be more natural light in the classrooms and that when looking up and through the windows one would see the treetops. Arun said the windows needed to be a certain height from the ceiling and the ground and a certain distance from one another. He said that if they wanted to build another altar it needed to face a particular direction. The altar could be simple or not—what mattered was that it was well maintained and never collected dust and that the bathroom was at least a minimum distance away from the altar. Arun said they should paint the walls two tones so that the top half was slightly lighter than the bottom half. He said they should place, under the central window, a potted plant that flowered with leaves and to set it on a piece of cloth that held sentimental value. Even if the cloth had holes in it, that would be fine, as that would only point further to the inescapable fragility and impermanence observed and experienced in life.

As Arun was speaking one could tell he was thinking about what he was saying and then, while laughing softly, he pointed to the hole in his own shirt as if some sort of poetic proof. He said a plant that flowered would cause people to pause, look, notice, and take in, and that those forms of reflection were needed to create balance within the constant flow of activity. He said it was important to love what one noticed.

Arun shared many little details with Sun and Das. He was encouraging about what the results would be. He said to see a vision one had to look for it in the particulars. Sun and Das agreed to follow his sage-like words as best as they could. Arun said that in the years to come they would all understand the meaning of such manifestations. All that Arun had said made sense to Sun and Das. He answered their questions in the way one sometimes feels one's questions are answered when speaking out loud to oneself. When questions come from a place of inquiry rather than worry, clutter, or conditioning, the answers will reflect that depth of wonder. Sun and Das thanked him for his insights, time, and thoroughness.

Arun and Clara remained friends throughout their lives. Arun liked Theo, and Clara liked Arun's wife, and often they'd come together to share their love for Indian food and spiritual conversation. There was one incident where Arun actually saved Clara from deep despair. Clara thought someone was trying to hurt her, and just when she was most convinced of it, she had a dream. In the dream she was sitting with a man in a simple rectangular building made from cinder blocks. In the dream she knew the man to be Arun's father. The room inside where they sat on chairs low to the floor, face to face and close to each other, had nothing much in it and no special qualities except a small paper statue of a god. Which god it was didn't seem to matter in the dream. Yet it was understood that this god was a protector, subtle, cosmic and supernatural, of this universe and beyond, and that on account of this dream, Clara knew that no one could harm her. Upon telling this to Arun, they were both relieved, as they were both aware that knowledge is received in the dreams of those who are attentive. Clara and Arun would often silently slip off into different worlds, where others and their ideas would appear to them with messages from elsewhere.

For Clara, Arun's father's dream building (its shape, its emptiness, its spaciousness, standing in the middle of nowhere, belonging to no one, anyone, and/or everyone), as she loosely described it—in the way one remembers, recalls, respects and retells one's dreams (telling them as they're dissipating, slipping away)—communicated all the necessary signs and symbols that could be seen as significant. She read and held them as seeds that would expand into gardens where she would continue to be serene.

Eli

Even though Eli would never have admitted it, he was a religious man. Perhaps he wouldn't admit it because he'd lived through a war where people were killed because they were religious. Or perhaps it was because he didn't speak much in general, and kept things to himself. Or perhaps Clara considered him religious, but he didn't think of himself in that way at all. For most of his life, he went to services at the temple once a week on Sabbath as well as special holidays. He was unassuming and stayed in the background but could never remain there, as people always noticed him.

During these services, the congregation or community of worshippers were frequently asked to "rise," which meant to stand, and then eventually "be seated." At certain times it was appropriate to stand and at other times to sit, and this etiquette was important to the rabbi, the congregation, and Eli. As Eli became old and fragile, this way of showing respect became quite difficult, for it was harder and harder for him to go from sitting to standing and back to sitting. Of course, many elderly people within the congregation also found this part of the service difficult. They chose to remain seated the entire time and this was considered perfectly acceptable. It was understood that it was not out of disrespect that these men and women stayed seated.

But Eli decided that if he couldn't stand up, he would stop attending the services. His family—Sarah, Solon, Esther, Clara, and Theo—all tried to convince him that he should still go, but he had made up his mind. Later, after he passed, Clara remembered that her father wouldn't sit in the temple while others stood, and though she couldn't quite put it into words she understood her father's decision. For her father, it was a form of letting go, an unburdening that revealed a larger dimension of her father that Clara had not been previously aware of. This dimension was made up of all the details of her father's life. Nothing was insignificant. His socks, shoes, metal arches, and ace bandages contributed to Clara's perceptions of her father and to his inability to stand and to accept his inability to stand if or when he attended services.

After Eli's passing, Clara looked for him in his shirts, his sweater, her pictures, in Sarah and Solon, even in Vienna. But he was absent and far away. She was afraid that he had disappeared completely from her life, as she couldn't see him anywhere. She decided to stop focusing so much on him and instead turned her attention to her mother. Clara knew that her father would have wanted this, for it had been her mother who had held the family together and had taken care of Eli in the last years of his life: when he could no longer stand up in the temple; when he was house-bound and lived on crackers and oranges, until he exploded one day and yelled at her for always giving him crackers and oranges when up to that point that was all he'd specifically asked for. Then he would say, "I want broccoli, only broccoli." Then after some time, it switched, and all he wanted was vanilla ice cream and grapes.

One time, when Clara was visiting her parents, Eli asked Clara to go to the store and buy him some grapes. He insisted on paying for them and gave her $2, which in Southern California at that time would have purchased perhaps ten grapes. He did not know how expensive grapes had become, especially the organic grapes that Clara bought that day, and it was good that he did not know. But later, after Eli passed and Sarah lived alone, Clara brought not grapes but bread and flowers to her mother, even though her mother always said, "Please don't bring anything." The day after such a visit Sarah would call and give thanks for the bread, which because it was a hundred percent rye reminded her of her childhood in Berlin; and for the flowers, which reminded her of Van Gogh and his sad story.

Clara enjoyed her visits with her mother, hearing stories about her childhood and noble family. When Clara and Theo visited, Sarah would wear her jewels and was illuminated by them. These jewels were cherished and had stories behind them of family, war, and love. Focusing on her mother made Clara happy and it was through this expression of love for her mother that her sorrow over her father diminished. Each time she took Sarah to the doctor, filled her mother's car with gas, helped her out of the bathtub, or sat next to her on the couch, she knew that Eli would be pleased, and somehow in pleasing him she felt his presence there and everywhere. Thus, there was a merger between Clara and her father, and the love for her father continued to grow even after he passed. Every elderly man she saw, and every father she saw, she loved.

Ling and Howard

It turned out that although Clara and Theo lived in a secluded area in a cabin at the foot of the mountain, they did have neighbors. The house of these neighbors was far enough away that Clara couldn't see it, but close enough to walk over. So it was comforting to be away from others on the one hand, but near others on the other. Ling and her husband Howard made wonderful neighbors. Ling loved to meditate and Howard, who did not meditate, built her a yurt to meditate in, separate from the house. Clara, Theo, and Ling sat together regularly in this yurt. Ling thought of herself as a beginner but was not. She was an old soul who was often in deep states of meditation. This was true whether she was formally sitting; or gardening; planting seeds and growing flowers and vegetables in the summer; or keeping the fire going, chopping wood, and picking up kindling or shoveling snow in the winter. She was mindful in her activities and so aware of her surroundings that she blended in, like a figure mistaken for a tree in a landscape in a Chinese ink drawing.

Clara would often wonder on her way to the yurt how it came to be that Ling was her neighbor. How was it that in her life there was now this yurt and a neighbor who loved to meditate? How did such things fall into place? Were there explanations? She would often think of someone and then they would telephone or appear. If she were traveling in an airplane she would be seated next to a priest, a rabbi, or a traveler on a pilgrimage, which to her was auspicious. Sometimes when she went to a restaurant, through talking with the waitress she would realize they had met before or had a mutual friend or a common obscure interest, like the novels of May Sarton or Henry Fox Talbot's photograms. She would go for a walk and just then a rainbow would appear; or she would stay inside and just when she looked out the window she'd see two bears or a red bird. She marveled at this river of unexplained moments and wondered where they came from . . . heaven? Earth? She trusted these experiences and as a result never felt the need to force things.

Sarah

Sarah had thought that when or if Eli passed before her, her life would be empty without him. As it turned out, she went to live near Clara in a retirement community center full of people like herself, in that they'd lived long lives and many of them had outlived a partner. She found herself at home in this place and made many new friends and especially enjoyed the dinners that were served there. She had grown so accustomed to simple and quiet meals with Eli that this change of having dinner with a group of others, accompanied by a bottle of wine, was welcome. Sometimes on the phone she'd describe to Clara the evening dessert (some kind of black forest cake or fruit cup with ice cream, something spongy, heavy, creamy, rich, tart . . .), for Eli had only liked applesauce. Sometimes Sarah would gather with her new friends and they would read plays; so she found herself reading the part of a character from Shakespeare or Chekhov or Shaw. In the reading of these plays, Sarah was able for a time to put her own thoughts aside and via the words pass from one reality to another.

Clara

As Clara took her seat on the train while traveling through Europe, she wondered if it was really heading where she wanted to go. She wondered which way the train was going and whether the direction of her seat was such that she would be riding forward or backward. She was hoping it would be forward but she was too worn out and tired to ask in a language unknown to her, so she decided to just wait and see.

The day before had been Wise One's birthday and it was the first time the birthday was celebrated since his passing. Friends of Clara's were spending time with Wise One's family and sending messages to Clara about the celebrations. These messages were flooding Clara with memories and these memories gave everything special meaning. She wanted to dwell on her memories, but the lady sitting across from her from Croatia wanted to talk to her or perhaps with anyone, so at last Clara surrendered her recollections to converse with the blond lady who seemed lonely and talkative. Clara remembered the many times in her life when she had been lonely, but she had not been talkative. Rather, she would close in on herself; just saying a few words, even if they were necessary, was painful.

So Clara's memories traveled from Wise One to her past lonelinesses, which even included her accident and her hospitalization; for the Croatian lady mentioned, within a few minutes of their conversation, that she had been hit in the head by a speedboat and that it had done a lot of damage. Eventually, the lady sat back and fell asleep, after being kind enough to switch directions with Clara (for Clara was in fact facing backward and very happy to switch directions), and after that decided to rest her mind and spend the rest of the journey looking out the window. Letting go of her memories, Clara enjoyed the train ride. She looked at the various shades of green around her: fields of flowers here and there; farms; rows of lettuces; houses that looked old, like they had been there for a long time, and she wondered about the people who lived and had lived in them. The houses, flowers, trees, and mountains shone at Clara as she simply observed them from the windows of her moving train.

In no time at all, the memories came back. The flowers reminded Clara of Theo's mother, Frances, who came from the mountains of Italy and still had a few pressed flowers that had been in the pages of a hard-cover book for decades and from time to time she'd take them out to look at. The houses reminded her of a quality of life that she assumed to be more spacious than living in an apartment: houses with windows all around, terraces, balconies, porches, front and back doors. The variety of greens reminded her of Van Gogh, and she felt grateful to know of him and his paintings. The tunnels reminded her of her soul and the journey it was taking from darkness to light. So it seemed that memories can fade, but not entirely or not for long; but as the memories went from the things of the world to her soul, she felt peaceful.

When Clara arrived at her destination, the first place she went to was the rose garden. She walked through the old city and the town square, stopped inside the church and sat for a while. She looked at the stained-glass windows and appreciated the views of the trees outside through a small open window. She looked at the votive candles, the wooden chairs, and hardcover books. She entered through the main door but left from a small side door, which led to a narrow flight of deep steps that she descended. At the bottom, she arrived at the river and the bridge, which she crossed over. This led to a path, uphill, which led to the famous rose garden. From the rose garden one could see the city, its rooftops and steeples.

Walking among the rose bushes, Clara felt affection for each bush. Each flower and every petal had something to explain in detail to her. Passing from one bush to another, she remained still in the movements of her mind. Signs next to each bush described each flower, but she renounced these signs and communicated with the flowers directly. The names of the flowers weren't important to her, at least in their presence; she wanted to look at them with as few thought processes as possible. Without her own thoughts she felt her mind more as a field and related it to the fertile ground within which the seeds of the rose bushes had originally been planted.

She wondered how the land had been tended to and how long it had been since the original planting of those seeds to the time when the seeds had flowered, and how many times they had flowered and for how long. She wondered about the gardener and if she or he would see a part of her- or himself in the rose, the way in which it blossomed and its beauty, for the gardener who had tended to the rose's cultivation understood its root systems. Questions about seeds and their relationships to their flowers were in her mind and she wondered about seeds in their abstractions: seeds to understanding; seeds that could be planted that would sprout and give new seeds that would replace the previous seeds that would eventually open; seeds that held hidden qualities, that would come as the result of the precious work that would make up her life.

Sun and Das

Sun's rose garden started out as a present of fifty bushes that a friend of hers had gifted to her for her fiftieth birthday. Sun planted the bushes herself, digging each hole two feet deep; as in everything she did, the flowers bloomed. Sun and Das never used chemicals in their gardens. Das had learned the old ways of the land and shared them with the local mountain people. Without Das ever saying anything, the mountain people trusted him, which was unusual since Das had come from the city and was not a local person. But Das was gentle and flower-like himself. Sometimes it was hard to know what gender he was. He seemed a primary being—elemental, naked, shining, and approachable.

Many characteristics made him distinct: his thinness, long hair, and tattoos; the jewelry he wore for over thirty years, which he never changed and which seemed symbolic rather than decorative; the mugwort wrappings around his feet, his gnarly veins, and the transparency of his skin. Yet these distinctions, which for most people would have dominated, did not stand out. He was so relaxed in his own mind and not preoccupied with external appearances that others in his presence were less likely to focus on differentiations, so that when they left him, their minds were less fractured.

It, therefore, made sense that these rose bushes were present to offer insights into the visible and invisible worlds as one took in the roses, first as concrete objects with names and then gradually as shapes and forms without names, and subtler still, simple and unmarked like a grain. Over time, the rose bushes of Sun and Das became as glorious and famous as the rose gardens that Clara had visited in Europe. The difference was that the bushes of Sun and Das weren't in rows or organized in a way that insisted on pattern. There was no gap between the gardener and the roses. The questions that Das had asked of the roses had had their importance, but then there was no longer any need for questions, as inquiries lead to answers and answers accumulate, and Das and Sun were not searching for answers or accumulations. Instead, their life would unfold, carry, lift, spread, envelop, and support.

Wise One

Wise One had been the support for so many and the source of so much good. But when Wise One passed and was empty of form, his purpose still remained and many felt him as a formless one. Wise One's divinity decorated all he no longer held onto. He was released of object-ness, but his supreme spirit was experienced even more as it was recognized as part of those who had known him, and even those who didn't. Sacredness flowed underneath the changing nature of life and this was a reflection of Wise One in the lucidity of the empty space, available to the ones with clear minds who could perceive this in the atmosphere. Accepting the passing of Wise One brought an appreciation for what passes and an acceptance of impermanence. This acceptance became a support, which replaced other supports, and was as simple as fresh air.

Like the signs that named the roses told something of the rose that the rose in and of itself could tell better, the formless Wise One answered all questions once all questions stopped being asked, soon after his physical form disappeared and went back to ash and into water. In this way, Clara, or Sun and Das, or anyone who had known and therefore missed Wise One, at times awoke from their sleep to find that during the night a bouquet of flowers had mysteriously been left in a vase on a table. How this had come to be could not be questioned or argued over. Themes around these flowers were given as well as meanings, but these themes and meanings took one away from the themes and meanings that could not be explained. The fragrance of these flowers could not be explained either. It could be described, even remembered, but the impressions left from the fragrance of these flowers that mysteriously appeared in the lives of so many in the middle of the night released them from misconceptions about themselves, who lived in the room next door, and the messages they brought.

BOOK II: Practice

Lucy

As Clara's life changed, one friend named Lucy always remained close. Lucy had come to New York City when she was seventeen to dance with a well-known company. She danced eighteen hours every day of the week. At a certain point, however, the work became arduous and Lucy felt that what began as voluntary had become something she did begrudgingly; at that point, she left the company. Her aspirations had changed. Still, Lucy wanted to find and dedicate herself to a discipline that would transform and guide her toward her highest potential. She knew that in order to do that it would have to be voluntary.

Clara was teaching yoga at the school that Sun and Das had created on the east side of New York City and one day Lucy in her search came to one of Clara's classes. Clara liked Lucy from the start. Lucy was graceful, with a tinge of awkwardness. She was gorgeous, had long thin arms and black hair, and wore black rectangular eyeglasses. After she stopped dancing, she worked as a fashion model and as part of her payment got to keep some of the clothes. She had a way of mixing the clothes she modeled with the clothes she bought, mostly second-hand, that Clara appreciated, and Lucy appreciated Clara's appreciation.

One day after Clara's class, they went for tea and that was the beginning of a long and wonderful relationship. Clara was surprised that Lucy had given up her career as a dancer. She was also surprised that Lucy, as beautiful as she was, was unhappy. Lucy lived in an apartment where the atmosphere was heavy with negativity and tension. Though it was their first time out together, Lucy told Clara many personal things and Clara listened well. At the end of their meeting, Clara, who lived alone, asked Lucy if she would want to live with her. Lucy agreed, and the two young women set out on a spiritual path together as lifelong friends, where they would for many years strive to reach their highest potential.

Many years later, when neither Clara nor Lucy lived anymore in Manhattan, Lucy fell in love with Vincent. Vincent had decided even before meeting Lucy that he, too, was on a path of transformation and believed that if he worked hard enough he could turn himself into an angel. He taught meditation to young men in trouble, in prison, or in reform schools. His own dark past enabled him to relate to these men and they to him. He was poorly paid for his work and lived on next to nothing, which was fine with him as the activities he most liked to do—meditate and pray—didn't require much money. He prayed for the welfare of all beings and had a particular way of sitting and praying that was practiced in ancient times. He had been taught these practices by a lama whom he met in Tibet. The practice was secret, quietly passed on, and not spoken of outside of the teacher and student. What Vincent could share with others was that each time he finished praying he washed his hands, and that the water he washed his hands with would carry the prayers far.

Lucy loved Vincent and even though she got angry with him for eventually going off into a cave to pray for three years in solitude and silence, her anger did not diminish her love: it increased it. She knew that through this labor and discipline Vincent would burn away his impurities, whatever they were, and replace them with learning. He could accept pain and welcome challenges and live on the edge, and Lucy knew that the degree to which he had these qualities and abilities exceeded ordinary limits. For these reasons, she waited three years for his return. She knew that neither of them could know beforehand the extent of the transformation that lay ahead, and she knew that he would suffer pain again and again voluntarily if he thought it would illuminate him.

Vincent did not have many books in his cave, but the few he had were scriptures and he studied them well. He contemplated what he read while learning about himself, and wondered how to incorporate the scriptures into his life. Because he was away from his teachers, he relied a good deal on his books. Even though he was not sitting at his teacher's feet as he so often had, he often felt while alone in his cave that he was receiving transmissions from them, and that the transmissions would remain with him forever, wherever he went in the world.

Vincent was only allowed one visitor and that was his lama, Lama Daniel. The lama could come three times a year to give guidance. Part of the reason for Vincent's retreat was that his lama, whom he loved, had gone on such retreats and Vincent wanted to follow in the footsteps of his lama. Vincent learned from Lama Daniel that the suffering in the world could be lessened if people listened to a guiding principle that lives everywhere, but is more easily accessed through the gradual purification of one's mind.

Vincent hoped that through his work in the cave he would put all of his excuses aside, giving himself the best chance to surrender and offer his life to this guiding principle. His surrender and humility lent a mood of freedom to his demanding retreat, which was also voluntary. Vincent did not go out of his way to make things easy for himself. On the contrary, the retreat was in a region of the country where summers are extremely hot and winters extremely cold, and his cave was a long hike up a steep hill. He experienced wind, hail, thunder, and lightning of biblical proportions. Yet he remained happy: happier than he had ever been or thought possible.

As time passed, Vincent was transforming. What was going on in his mind no one could know, but when his lama came to visit he saw that Vincent was happier. Vincent's cave was small, his window small, but his view of the desert, rocks, and mountains was far-reaching. He enjoyed this dichotomy. In his cave, looking out into the vast space, he experienced single-pointed focus. Prior to the retreat, he had read poems about the ocean, its waves and tides, and the mood of focus its vastness could inspire. He now understood these poems when he looked out of his cave at the desert rocks and mountains.

This newfound ability to focus and the calm it brought him was what Lama Daniel perceived in Vincent. A coating, a covering, an obscurity had been removed and Vincent was quite literally lighter. It was a level of concentration that Vincent experienced in his meditations, of the land through his window, that he had been looking for. Vincent thought often about the Buddha, as he knew the Buddha had experienced high levels of concentration. What he knew of Buddhism was that God or no God, the eternal spirit, nothing or everything, was realized only if and when one could concentrate. Distractions had to stop. That was the reason for his retreat. Leaving the world, he thought, would help him to leave his distractions, and he was right; it did, for a time. He could see mankind in the desert flower and its deterioration: its inevitable death, its return to the earth, its silence, its end. And yet, because his mind was empty he could see something of the flower that would live on, and be even more far-reaching than his view.

Frances

In her nineties, Frances had also become lighter. Like Vincent, she'd left the pushing and pulling of the world, though not so much out of choice: she had been forced to, as she had grown frail with age. She was afraid, rightly so, to leave her apartment: that the wind would blow her down, or the people run her over, or that she'd lose her way. So her apartment became like a cave. But because the neglected back yard was so overgrown and so much new building had occurred, with high-rises all around, she had no view from her window. Her view was of truth itself. She could see everything without opening her eyes. She had become a philosopher, and her dwelling a refuge.

She had theories for why people suffered, and these theories, which she was humble about, were born out of a knowledge that was the outcome of a long hard life, which had always included inquiry. Frances's questions, her simple way of life, her ability to save money, and the time she had at the end of her life for pondering, revealed many truths to her. She realized that she had made herself suffer and saw this, too, in everyone around her: patterns of behavior that were destructive and repeated. She referred to this as ignorance, the inability to see how and why we cause ourselves to suffer. She knew this ignorance came from mistaking the unreal for the real, the untruth for the truth, and the impermanent for the permanent. It was and is the great delusion: that we are undivine. There was some common ground or universal feeling that people were cut off from. It is why people have been and are killing each other in wars. It makes people hard and uncaring. It was, as Frances saw it, a darkness, fertile: like a field where many dangerous seeds could easily sprout over and over again.

Since Frances no longer left her apartment, her children visited her. During these visits Frances spoke of her theories, and her children knew that it was here, in the viewless apartment, surrounded by a collection of things of no value except to her, that a real treasure was: a person with depth who had been exploring the nature of the Self for decades, with exceptional wisdom, without having had any formal education except life itself and curiosity.

Whenever the children came for short or long visits they were touched by Frances's knowledge and reminded of something forgotten, which Frances refused to give a name to, for she felt that words could only diminish and mislead. In addition to the children visiting, were the strangers whom Frances let in from the street to help her. Sometimes these strangers would return and sometimes not. A nurse from an agency came to teach Frances how to use a walker and how to bathe in a chair. There were also friends of her children who lived nearby and would come over, especially if her children were traveling, to bring Frances the newspaper, and fruit if it was summer.

Frances had a theory that people with a high opinion of themselves, who thought they were superior, suffered just as much as those with a low opinion of themselves, who thought they were inferior. She said people were all the same. Wise One had said the same thing, and so actually did the Buddha. But almost everyone flips from one to the other—too good or not good enough—and because of this people were jealous and afraid of one another. Frances said that often when people felt inadequate they bought things or in some way consumed: all the time wanting something, caught in a cycle of desires that would never end because the cause of the craving was this wrong view of oneself. She said that when people were bothered or uncomfortable it was because they didn't like themselves, that people had turned what they didn't like about themselves outward and somehow were projecting it onto their world. She said that this was why people had become greedy: that they had lost a sense of their inner worth, their common ground.

Frances said that when she was younger she had not known these things, that she had always compared herself to others, and that it had only been in the last ten years of her life that many of her questions or confusions had cleared up. For this, she was grateful to have lived so long. At the same time, she was not afraid to die. In her own way, she was preparing, organizing her closets and drawers, as if she was going on a long trip. She answered her unanswered letters, forgave her mother, tried to understand her father, made peace with her children, wrote down her thoughts and theories, and read Dante. She did not feel fearful or doomed, neither in life nor in death. She took rest in her epiphanies, what she had come to know, how she had educated herself, and all that she had noticed, reconciled, and loved. When she was near to her death she said that after her death she would be able to oversee everything and that she would understand all she had not been able to understand while limited to being in a body. She said that after her death she could always be reached; if anyone wanted to reach her, she would travel in the breezes through the air or the rays of the sun or in infinite other ways. She assured her children not to worry.

Unlike Frances, Clara did fear death. Perhaps it wasn't death that she feared so much as loss. She was afraid of being bitten by dogs or struck by lightning. She worried about fires to the extent that she did not burn candles or incense and was constantly checking the stove. She feared that one of her cats might eat a poisonous flower or be eaten by a predator; she would have liked to keep her cats indoors, but they both loved the outdoors so much it seemed unfair to withhold that experience from them. There were a few people she was afraid she might disappoint so that when she was in their presence she was nervous and would not be herself, except for those times when she could be herself and felt her fear go away.

Was life a waiting room, an entrance, an ingress before one was forced into an inevitable end? Would this end be a transmission, a change into a new dwelling made easier through a process of letting go? Did one simply dissolve? Was there something left? Was the body a house of desires and insecurities, a container for light, or both?

Vivian

Clara had a friend called Vivian, who seemed to approach life as if everything was happening for the first time. If she had a banana on the table turning from green to yellow she would say, "Did you see the banana lately? It's half green and half yellow." Even though Vivian had seen this happen before, the fulfillment she felt through seeing the banana skin change colors was not diminished because of it. This was one of many reasons why Clara liked hanging out with Vivian. The past did not obscure Vivian's vision of the present. This rare and exalted state came naturally to her. As a result, she was often laughing or crying over the beauty or wondrousness of some aspect of life that might have been considered commonplace by others.

Vivian studied Asian poetry in college and afterwards wrote two books of poems in haiku style. These books, describing the wonders of mundane objects, were successful, so that after the sales of the second book she had saved some money (rare for a poet) and with those savings decided to leave New York City to start a new chapter in her life elsewhere. This move was also instigated by a failed relationship, in which her lover left her without any explanation or forewarning the day before their planned wedding. This experience devastated Vivian to such a degree that she felt it best to move to Australia, literally the other side of the world. All of this had happened when she was twenty-three, long before she met Clara in India where they shared an apartment while studying with Wise One. In a rare moment of disclosure as they waited for a bus late at night, when people sometimes say things they otherwise wouldn't, Vivian told

Clara her story. In fact, Vivian's real name wasn't even Vivian; what it was she did not say.

Because, despite their time together in India, the two women lived so far from each other, and because Clara did travel a lot sometimes, when Clara was traveling and somewhere in between the U.S. and Australia (but closer to Australia), Vivian would make a trip to meet her. Thus, they grew accustomed to looking for each other in airports and bus or train stations, crowded with people and languages they did not know. Often there would be a space of one to two years between such visits and Clara would anticipate what Vivian would be like. On the last of such visits, at an airport in a polluted noisy city, upon their meeting Clara almost did not recognize Vivian. Her hair, which was thick and had always been remarkably long and shiny, was short but not styled, and looked as if it had been cut in some kind of rage or attack on herself. The hair had also lost its radiance. This decline in the appearance of her dear friend's hair told Clara many things that had nothing to do with hair, and Vivian could see in her friend's eyes a shock and recognition of something that hopefully they could speak of—that had been and still was painful.

Since the last time they had met, Vivian had fallen in love, at the age of fifty. Up to that point she'd had very little romantic experience outside of her great disappointment as a young woman. After that, it had been hard for her to be close to anyone, so she thought she would remain alone for the rest of her life. Then when she least expected it, at the wedding of her eldest brother's son, she had met a good friend of her brother's, whom she had known in her youth but had not seen in many years. This man had never married, as he was happy living with and taking care of his parents while earning a small living making dandelion wine. Vivian appreciated his humility while he appreciated the mystery of her sadness. One thing led to another and it seemed to both of them that they had each found in the other their soul mate. Then, after only a few months, the happiest that Vivian had perhaps ever known, the man while walking through the woods was mistakenly shot dead by a hunter. Upon the tragic news, Vivian went into hiding. For more than a year no one knew anything of her whereabouts. When she finally emerged, she cut her hair. It was the most poignant way at that time for her to reconcile herself to her loss.

The night that Clara and Vivian shared was different than the others in that though Vivian had booked her own hotel room she ended up staying with Clara. Vivian wanted to speak of her tragedy, but when Clara asked how she had been she said nothing but waved her hands in front of her, recreating the blockade that she'd remained behind for much of her life. Clara sensed that she had maybe probed too far, too fast, and regretted it. At the same time, she felt that if nothing was said this would somehow create a barrier as well, the absence of truth.

Honey, Juniper, and Hazel

Clara had had cats all her life. When she and Theo moved into their cabin, the previous owner left behind two kittens. He and his wife had so many cats that Clara and Theo thought they might have accidentally "forgotten" these two. They were lying in a box upstairs, one on top of the other. Clara named one Honey and Theo named the other Juniper. Honey and Juniper were sisters. Clara took the kittens as a sign that she and Theo were meant to leave the city and move to the cabin in the woods. She had never seen two cats care for each other the way that Honey and Juniper did. They were together all the time.

One day when the cats were playing, Juniper scratched Honey on her nose. Time passed, but a scar remained, and Clara wished the scar would fade. At the age of three, Juniper unexpectedly died. After Juniper's death, Clara hoped that the scar on Honey's nose would remain. When she looked at it, she traced it back to Juniper. Months after Juniper's passing, an abandoned and wild cat appeared in view of the cabin. When Clara approached the seemingly young cat, the cat ran away, but appeared again the next day. Each day she appeared and each day she ran off, but less and less far until after a couple of weeks she stayed and followed Clara into the cabin. Theo and Clara named her Hazel because of the color of her eyes. Honey and Hazel did not care for each other the way that Honey and Juniper had; but in some way it seemed good that they had each other. Hazel had orange and black fur that got matted because it was so long.

Having come in from the outside, Hazel appreciated her new home. But it would take time for her to trust in the kindnesses that her new surroundings offered. During this time she was always scared that someone, person or animal, would take her food or her place. She was unsure as to when or whether things would change and was unsettled. However, through the routine of breakfast and dinner and the consistent love and affection she received, Hazel changed. The worries and fears, real to her in her cat's body, eventually ended. Once her anxieties passed and she was free to be herself, she would lay for hours on the windowsill watching the goings-on outdoors: the weather, the wildlife, the insects, and the winds. The more she watched from her support, the more her body expressed a growing faith in her new life.

Gita

When Clara was in India she studied singing with Mr. Chandra, a music teacher who lived with his wife and two children in Sarana. Mr. Chandra's parents had both been musicians and all the members of his extended family, including his wife, were musical. When Mr. Chandra was busy, one of his relatives would teach for him. Because of this, Clara studied with many of his relatives and learned different skills from each one. Mostly though, as it turned out, she studied with his daughter Gita. When these lessons began Gita was only fourteen and Clara was forty-three—old enough to be her mother. In fact, Clara was older than Mr. Chandra, but always forgot, probably because he was her teacher, but also because he had aged differently from her and looked older. He aged when he lost his job, was diagnosed with diabetes, and found out that the owner of the lovely house where he and his family were living was returning, so that within a few months he would have to relocate his family to a slum in Bangalore.

It was clear that Gita was gifted musically. Everyone said that she must have been a great musician in a past life and for that reason chose to be born into the Chandra family. When she was young, her parents asked her to clean the altar, and while she cleaned she sang. Later, when she was much older, she said that cleaning the altar as a child had made a great impression on her.

Clara wondered about the circumstances of her own life as well as that of Gita's. What had she done to warrant such good fortune to have Gita for her music teacher? What determined the particulars of her birth, her family, teachers she had studied with, the condition of her health? Why was it that she always had food, medicine, clothes, and books that she needed and wanted? Why did Gita and her family have to leave the house and city they liked and move to a place they didn't, where the air was hard to breathe? Why did Mr. Chandra have poor health and why did his students typically not have money such that he could not charge enough for his lessons to live somewhere that he and his family liked? Why was it that Gita had a singing voice that was not talked of or even known about within the circles of prominent musicians in India, even though the quality and purity of her voice far exceeded most of the other singers?

Through her observations of nature, Clara had seen seeds sprout and flower. She knew that external conditions would determine how well this would occur. She came to think that her actions and the actions of others made impressions that acted as seeds planted in the minds, stomachs, cells, tissues, chambers, mansions, and storehouses of herself and others. She believed that the fields she observed in which weeds and flowers grew were no different from her internal fields, and that through time and conditions the seeds of her past actions would inevitably bear fruit and cause the quality and circumstances of her future. She understood that it took time for seeds to sprout. Around her cabin were trees that were several hundred years old. The leaves on these trees had changed color and fallen many times. The seeds of the fruits had been carried elsewhere by the winds and the birds, and with those winds and birds came the collective creation of new trees. As time passed, the trees would grow large, as the seeds in the fertile fields of Clara's mind would also, and she realized that in creation everyone was a gardener.

On the day that Clara, in Sarana, had her first lesson with Gita, who at fourteen sung so beautifully and delivered her lesson so well, Clara pondered what seed she could have planted in her mind to cause this blessing. Clara thought of the teachings she had given, the songs she had taught, her love for music, and her ability to listen for long periods of time to symphonies and operas.

Clara had a friend named Alana who adopted a boy from a village in Africa. The boy's mother had died of a terrible disease and his father thought the child would have a better life with a mother, even if not a blood mother, in a country where he believed there were less terrible diseases and more general stability. Alana was told that the boy was five years old, but when she picked him up in Africa he seemed more like eight.

When the boy first got to America, it was difficult for him to make friends. Alana thought he was musical because he sung in the shower songs that he had grown up with in his village, and she did not want him to forget these songs. The two of them lived simply on her small income from cleaning people's houses. One day, Clara put some money in Alana's purse with a note, *So your son can have music lessons.* Alana looked for a teacher for her son. She contacted a church in Brooklyn where the congregation was international—with men, women, and families from different parts of Africa, even some from the region where her son had been born.

She found among them an older man who came from the same small village as her adopted son, who knew all the same songs, plus many more. This man was part of a group from the congregation that came to gather together in the basement of the church once a week to sing their native songs. Alana's son was welcomed into the community and this was the beginning of his feeling at home in New York City and in the world as well. The songs included descriptions of the four seasons that move with the sun, moon, and stars; of the skies in the mornings of cold days in winter; or of long afternoons of summer that praised and celebrated life. Even sad songs—ballads of heroes and heroines starving for food, love, or both—when set to song were uplifting. These were wisdom songs that flow underneath the surfaces of ignorance, and Alana couldn't quite believe how amazing her son was, especially when he was singing, or later when he was explaining to her their meaning, for many of the songs were not in English.

Clara pondered if it was because of this small amount of money she had put in Alana's purse more than a decade before that Gita was now teaching Clara songs. For Alana always said that had it not been for the note *So your son can have music lessons* she may have used the money differently and eventually her son may have forgotten these songs from his village and tried to fit in in other ways.

Over the years, a few of Clara's students went to study with Gita, and these students paid Gita exceptionally well. Gita gathered enough money from teaching to go to college. At the college she impressed everyone so much that immediately after graduation she was offered a job teaching at the college, and her income made it possible for the family to move again, but this time back to a nicer area.

Clara

Clara experienced joy and sorrow in her own life and in the lives of others and wanted to know the cause of joy and sorrow. This inquiry led her back to her garden, to the seeds she had planted and the flowers and vegetables she had watched grow. She trusted that if she planted a potato seed, she would get a potato. There was some certainty to it that she compared to mathematics or laws of gravity. There would be no apple as a result of planting a potato tuber. Clara found this reassuring and thought how difficult it would be to plant a seed and not know what type of fruit it would bear. She felt the relationship between seeds and their fruit was something important for her and others to understand. She thought of the joys and sorrows in her life as fruits and followed them back, within her mind, through her life, looking to locate their seeds.

Through her search, she understood more deeply the relationship to and process of planting what she wanted to see grow and sowing seeds of happiness. She thought these findings would be helpful in the way in which she might experience her future and improve her world at the seed level. She thought of how small a seed is, how forests had come from seeds, and how large the forests were, especially before they had been chopped down. She recalled photos she had seen from the nineteenth century of a person standing in a landscape and how large the trees or small the person appeared in contrast to the other. She pondered the type of mental seeds that were being planted and causing such present-day violence to the forests. She wondered why the violence to the animals and Earth was spreading so quickly. She wanted to take actions that would stop this violence and plant different kinds of mental seeds where animals and trees could live out their lives as peacefully as she and most people would want to.

There had been times in Clara's life when her sorrows took her to different places. She would leave one place where she felt sorrow for another. Many times she had done this. Sometimes this changing of places provided a change, a lift from sorrow; at other times she just brought her sorrows along, for they had become a part of her. They were too deep inside to disappear just by changing her environment on the outside. Changing things on the outside was like changing one's eyeglasses. Wise One used to say that one needed to change more than the eyeglasses one used to see with if one wanted to change the world one was seeing.

Gazelle

Through her travels, Clara had been to places where people were, so it seemed, less fortunate than she. This meant that basic needs, food, hygiene, shelter, and safety were not available. Of course, Sarah and Eli had gone through years without these basic needs, as well as Frances, on account of the war. But these were the elders, the mothers and fathers, and not those of Clara's generation; most people she knew of her age had not had such experiences.

Then one day, a young woman from a war-torn country, a princess of sorts named Gazelle, showed up in her class. Gazelle had golden hair, green eyes, and many freckles. She had frail arms and support braces around her wrists. She worked in the corporate world and had achieved a high level of success. She worked long hours, woke up early, went to bed late, and was well paid. The income she earned gave her plenty of money, which she bought things with: nice clothes, items for the apartment, and specialty foods, which she rarely ate because she dined out often. She traveled first class, stayed in expensive hotels, took taxis, tipped well, went for manicures and massages, and still had a significant amount of money left to send to her family back home.

She enjoyed her work and her pay, yet she questioned its value. She understood that to be a nurse or a firefighter had value, but wasn't sure about her job and the life she had built around it. This bothered her. What was it all for? She didn't see the corporation as necessarily serving others in a worthwhile way. This was on her mind when she came to Clara's class. She wasn't sure what to expect, but what she found changed her life completely. That night in class, Clara spoke on the anxiety of impermanence and change. She said that wisdom was seeing what underlies all that was in flux, and referred to this underlying, undying essence as the soul. She said that the soul was different from all that is in flux in that the soul is unchanging. She said that if we identified with our souls, we would worry less about our lives. Gazelle had not heard words used to describe the soul such as "un-entangled, pure, everlasting," in a long time, if ever. Gazelle sensed that the emptiness she felt in her life had something to do with what she was hearing.

After that talk, Gazelle came every week to class, and she and Clara became fast friends. Gazelle realized that there was a thin veil covering her soul and that that veil could be removed. She told Clara about her childhood, having to sleep in the hallway because the hallways were without windows and windows were targets for bombs. Clara told Gazelle that she had never looked at windows that way. Gazelle told Clara that if someone in her family went to the store, it was uncertain if they would return. She said that as a child she had played with children of the "other side," but as a young adult had grown distrustful. When she left her country to come to America, first as a student and later for work, she left her childhood experiences behind. She had not spoken about them in years and here she was confiding in Clara.

It was an unburdening, as she had not realized how weighed down she was by her memories. This unloading felt extraordinarily good.

Clara soon took Gazelle to meet Sun and Das and they were able to show Gazelle the way to end her sorrow. Gazelle had to learn how to garden. It was through sowing seeds and understanding how they sprout that she could change the way she was feeling. It was true that she had suffered a lot growing up, but this was suffering that had already happened. The teachings that Sun and Das shared contained practical and scientific methods to prevent suffering in the future. It didn't mean that everything would go as planned or exactly how Gazelle wanted. It didn't even mean that she would never experience war again. What it meant was that she would come to know that which was unchanging.

On account of Gazelle's childhood in a country that was often at war, with bombs thrown through windows and so many uncertainties, she wasn't spoiled and had a natural empathy toward everyone. Her happiness over someone else's happiness was so real that she almost needed no real happiness of her own.

Eventually, Gazelle left her job to study closely these new, but old, philosophies that addressed her soul. Her coworkers were sad to see her go. The head of her department offered her everything he could, but her purpose for being there had come to an end. She had earned enough money and sent enough of it home. She had enough clothes, perfume, and had had enough manicures and nice meals out. She had enjoyed the things of the senses but was not fulfilled by them. It was time to abandon this way of life.

Lama Daniel

Lama Daniel was a great fundraiser and had projects all over the world. He had developed an organization whose purpose was to save ancient books from being torn apart and sold page by page on the black market, or left to rot in unused libraries, by first buying the books himself.

Once the books were in his possession he hired people, usually women and usually refugees, to type the scriptures into a computer. He developed typefaces so that the old languages were retained in their original alphabets and succeeded in persuading the major computer companies in wealthier parts of the world to donate computers. Like this, he saved thousands of sacred books, tens of thousands of poetic verses, and even more ancient words, with infinite meanings, as well as providing dignified work for those forced out of their countries.

When he would talk about these projects—the books and their importance, the work and self-respect that the work saving, documenting, transcribing, and translating generated, and the monasteries and libraries where the books were later placed—inevitably Lama Daniel would cry. He was an emotional monk. Sometimes it took a long time to explain the progress or growth of a project, because of the intermittent crying. But time waiting for him to stop crying softened everyone's heart that needed softening from a harder reality that was rigid and dominated by dullness or agitation, and not the bright light that was shining in the holy books that Lama Daniel was in the act of preserving. He made everyone feel the importance of saving a book written centuries ago, that would then last many years into the immediate future and beyond, all the while enlightening the readers and caretakers of these books. He cherished books and inspired the reading of them.

Lama Daniel also raised money to send to monasteries to provide food for the monks in India, Tibet, Malaysia, China, Mexico, Russia, and Ethiopia, who without his funds would possibly have gone hungry. Some of the monks were not in their homeland as they'd been made to leave on account of their beliefs. They had walked for days, weeks, and months out of their country carrying whatever they could. They had gone without food or water through difficult terrain, where the weather was at times severe. They lost many of the men, women, and children they had originally started with, who could not withstand the journey or the pain of separation from the land of their ancestors, which they loved and thought of as home. Every monk that survived the journey was broken, with an illness and a tragic story. They eventually built new monasteries in new places and painted pictures of their home, its mountains and temples, on the walls. These paintings were colorful and depicted stories of the Buddha.

Bowls of fruit, vegetables, and nuts painted on painted altars, placed before painted gods on painted walls, in a painted temple of lands that were painted yet real for these monks. The suffering they had undergone in the loss of their country and most of their books was transformed through the painting. They had dreams of rainbows and painted those dreams in mandalas on the walls. The mandalas were an offering to anyone looking to end their sorrows. People came to visit the monasteries and were absorbed by the paintings and uplifted by the panorama of forms and colors surrounding them.

Lama Lothar

Lama Daniel sent Clara along with Lucy to one of these monasteries—not to see the paintings, though he knew they would love seeing them, but rather to deliver a large sum of money he'd raised for the monks to buy rice. It seemed to Lucy and Clara that they had arrived just in time, for everyone looked hungry and the vessels in the kitchen were almost empty. As soon as the two women explained that Lama Daniel had sent them, they were given an extraordinary welcome. A spirit of celebration and gratitude entered the atmosphere. Lucy and Clara were served tea and provided with a translator who took them to see the head lama so they could deliver the money they had brought with them.

To get to the quarters of Lama Lothar, the head abbot, it was necessary to walk on a path made of cut grass through a field of high grass. It was a hot day and Clara had forgotten her hat. The sun was strong and she started to feel weak. When she arrived at Lama Lothar's home, she needed to lie down immediately, which she did. Lama Lothar's attendant covered her with a light cover and all she wanted to do was sleep. When she awoke hours later, she felt much better. She was hungry and the monks had prepared a meal for her and Lucy of noodles with green chilies, so that had she not awoken herself soon, someone would have come and woken her.

During the meal, Lucy spoke of all she had seen while Clara had been sleeping, of the monastery and her visits with five of the highest and eldest monks. Lucy knew that it was on account of Lama Daniel that she was granted these visits and that otherwise she would never have had the opportunity of entering the homes of the abbot and these particular monks. Many of the monks in the monastery would have had to wait for long periods of time, if not forever, to have such visits. Lucy understood the rarity of this privilege and it affected her in a way that she could not put into words. Each monk she visited lived across the expanse of a field and had their own way of speaking to her of the elemental world, so that her mind was opened to new ways of discovering and understanding the nature of earth, air, fire, water, and space.

Lama Lothar had a small Tibetan woven rug, just large enough for him, Lucy, and Clara to sit on. After the meal, they sat down on the rug. Clara spoke about what it was like to travel carrying so much money that wasn't hers. She had kept the money in a small bag with a drawstring inside a larger bag with straps that buckled shut. The larger bag was a shoulder bag with a wide strap she had worn the entire time she'd been traveling, except when she slept and used the bag as a pillow. The bag itself was worn and unassuming, and she figured that no one would know how much money was inside, yet she still kept her eyes on it. She was, therefore, relieved to have arrived safely with all the money in hand. Lama Lothar listened to Clara's story and afterwards told her about the rug they were sitting on. His sister had made it. He said that she was clairvoyant and could see what most people could not. She lived alone in a landscape that was flat, where she could see far in all directions. The skies were blue and the winds warm and not many people lived in the area.

At first she was lonely, but then she started making rugs. After a few years, people came to see what she was doing and it turned out that the people who came received messages from the rugs, so it was believed that the rugs held spirits that contained codes that communicated threads of significance to those who could read them. Word spread, and many people arrived from all over to buy these rugs. People bought them for their homes and as gifts, sometimes for special people or public places like the lobby of Carnegie Hall, and often returned to buy another. They told their friends and the word traveled, so Lama Lothar's sister was surrounded by people who loved her rugs and who understood she was a great artist. People commissioned the rugs, but no one ever specified a design because it was known that she would always know best. His sister was no longer lonely and Lama Lothar said that she also sent money to the monastery that she received from the sale of her rugs; that actually she only kept a small percentage, enough to make the rugs and to survive on.

Lama Lothar said what interested him most about his sister's rugs was the reverse side, and to explain why to Lucy and Clara, he turned part of the rug over so it was showing. It was this side that revealed how the rug was made. The handwork and the up-down, over-and-back movement of the thread were more evident. Lama Lothar pointed out the knots, which he said revealed the skill that determined how long the rug would hold together, and that the knots in and of themselves were an art. He said that people who knew a lot about rugs would always look at the reverse side, but that ordinarily it is the front that captivates people. He said it is the back, the invisible side, that tells how the rug was created, and that the weaver is exposed more in the underside than the front.

What Clara liked most about the rug was its simplicity. It was only two colors: light blue and gold. The pattern was uncomplicated and the light blue and gold were vibrant next to each other. It had some slight imperfections, irregular rows and faded color here and there. But she thought that these imperfections enhanced the rug, and that had the pattern been more complicated the imperfections would have been less noticeable. She shared her thoughts with Lama Lothar and Lucy, and they understood.

Emmet

Emmet invited a small group of friends to his house in the middle of the summer when the moon was full and the crickets were singing songs. Since he did not use electricity, his guests, who were not used to sitting in relative darkness, appreciated the light of the moon as it came in through the windows. Clara ended up giving a small informal talk on the attraction of sorrow. She sat in a small rocking chair surrounded by candles. It was an ideal setting for such a talk and the atmosphere was peaceful. Emmet had placed four watermelons in a pile of hay that were later to be eaten and made an exquisite bouquet of wild flowers, which was placed on a table. How he put together this bouquet blind was hard to understand. Without sight, he saw. Perhaps he saw clearer than those with sight in that he wasn't distracted.

After Clara's talk, people stayed and the watermelon was cut open and eaten. Clara stepped outside and walked past the old oak trees, hydrangea bushes, and the wooden fence, turned around and went back inside the house, which was decaying. Clara peeked into Emmet's bedroom, for the door was half open, and saw that his bed was unmade. Even the rumpled and crumpled way that the old linens fell touched Clara, who had always made her bed, except immediately after her father died. On each side of his bed and at the end of the hallway were mirrors, for Emmet collected them, so that from where she stood everywhere she looked—either over at the half-made bed or down the candlelit corridor, or up the narrow and steep flight of stairs—she saw herself, and it felt as if the house and all Emmet's belongings were reflections of her.

Sun and Das

Every summer, Sun and Das opened their home and garden to their students and taught them about nature. It seemed it was a belief in society that nature was to be taken, like shells on the beach. Because of this, there were very few shells on beaches anymore. Sun and Das found fulfillment in living with nature, knowing that shells exist and seeing them when at the seashore. They felt that when that fulfillment was missed, when the moment to meditate on the seashell was lost, it turned to desire, the desire to take or control. They taught people how to go back to the moment where one appreciates the shell and to leave the shell alone, in its surroundings. That to leave without the shell would be more fulfilling than to leave having taken it.

Sun and Das communicated directly with the goddesses of nature and believed that it was because of them that the vegetables in their garden grew so well. People from all over the world came to be near them and around one another. Sun and Das's home and garden and the forest behind their home became a refuge not only for the animals, who otherwise would have been hunted and killed, but also for humans (also animals) who wanted to settle down in the depth of a deeper reality in harmony with nature.

Sarah

At the age of eighty-six, Sarah visited those who like herself were weak and old, and at times infirm, hospitalized, without appetite, without family, and close to death. These visits exhausted Sarah such that one night when arriving home she collapsed in her chair with the lights off and listened to the sound of pouring rain, as she did not have the strength to turn on the lights or get up and close the window. The rain was heavy and lasted only ten minutes, but then ten minutes later it started again. Sarah was unusual in that she visited and comforted anyone she had heard was suffering especially and did not limit these visits to friends, people she liked, or people who were like her. This meant that she had a large and varied circle of people whom she genuinely cared for who were in many ways politically, temperamentally, religiously, etc. different. She placed much less importance on externals than most people do. She had compassion for those who were suffering and didn't care if they were like her.

Kate

Around the corner from where Clara and Theo lived was a farm. It was run by a large family of seven brothers, their wives and children. At the height of summer, the busiest time of the season, even the nieces, nephews, and friends would come to help out. The farm was called KATE'S, named after the farmer's wife. Kate had long brown hair that she tied back, big brown eyes, and long eyelashes. She was tall and strong. She had long arms and long legs and moved each arm and leg in sync with the other when she was walking. One would often see her walking from the farm to the stand or the stand to her house or from her house to her mother's across the street. She always wore the same plain clothes that hung loosely on her tall long body, and Clara considered Kate much more attractive than she probably thought herself to be.

Kate was always at the farm stand. Clara bought all her vegetables there during the farming season, which was late May through late November. In this way, after many years of living in the city, Clara learned what was in season: berries came in June, broccoli in July, tomatoes in August, squash in September, pumpkin in October, and Brussels sprouts in November. Clara and Theo enjoyed eating what was in season. The rest of the year when the farm stand was closed they ate more grains—rice and millet, fewer vegetables, and almost no fruit at all until the following June when the farm stand reopened with berries. Kate was hard working. She had raised four kids, who all went to college. Her three sons studied the history of agriculture, as they were planning to be farmers, and the youngest, Kate's only daughter, studied nursing.

Clara loved going to the farm stand, and while there she often thought of Vincent's elaborate rituals concerning food, and Lucy, who had become a doctor and most of the time prescribed food as medicine and always kept a cucumber or garlic bulb on her altar. There was a reverence for food that Lucy and Vincent shared that Clara experienced at the farm stand. From the stand, you could see across the road the vegetables growing in the earth, and often when you bought a potato or carrot some dirt was still on it.

Many years before Clara was buying vegetables at the farm stand, a particular man, whom Kate mistrusted, was a regular customer at the stand. This man would often say horrible things about people with dark skin. He would tell jokes loud enough for everyone to hear that Kate did not find funny. He would say crude things, especially if men, women, and children with dark skin were there. When this happened, Kate would look down at the ground, avoiding eye contact with anyone, as it made her uncomfortable to have this taking place at her stand.

Years later, Kate told Clara that if that was to happen now she would say something and make it known that that was unacceptable at her stand. It was two decades later, but she still remembered and regretted it. It was these types of stories that she would share with Clara when she came to buy melon, cucumber, or corn. Clara always left with the feeling that Kate, who rarely left the farm, knew the purpose of life and that this purpose resonated in Kate, in the farm stand, and in all the fruits and vegetables she ate from there.

One summer, a terrible storm passed through the region of Kate's farm. This type of weather was unusual for this area. For several days it rained so heavily that it was considered dangerous to be out in the rain. The ground could not absorb the amount of rain, so the water levels climbed high on houses, flooding the insides. Rivers and creeks completely washed out the roads. For three days the sky was dark, winds were strong, many trees fell on houses and in the road, and many homes lost their electricity, which everyone was so used to and dependent on.

Kate's farm was devastated; heads of cabbage floated down the road, ruined. The whole crop was gone and that fall the farm stand had nothing to sell. Kate's husband had a worried look on his face, but she had a different way of looking at the change in their farm. Somehow, the destruction of their crop that year made her feel more love and compassion, not only for all that she had loved before but a wider love for anyone who had lost what they had worked hard for or who had failed at something—which was, when she thought about it, almost everyone at some time somewhere.

This shock gave Kate a greater awareness of others, including the insects who had dug holes in the ground on their farm to bury their eggs in, whom she'd never before considered with quite the same level of compassion or companionship as she did after the storm. Even though the farm had changed and there was no work now to do until the following spring when they could turn the soil again, and even though they kept the farm stand open with nothing to sell or pile into baskets or carry to people's cars, there was something that had not changed, and that was perhaps what spiritual seekers are and have always been seeking: the innermost, the unchanging. During that time, Kate glowed and her husband was in awe of her, as it was evident that she could weather and flow with the ups and downs of life gracefully. He had always known this to be true of his wife, but it seemed that throughout the flood the loss of their crop and the damage done to their home he witnessed a new level of consciousness in his wife that he had not seen before. He had watched her in a quiet calm, as the sky got black. He had seen in her eyes all that he had affection for. He realized that the storm and its harshness also contained lessons in subtle and immaterial ways. These lessons took him to a greater level of insight that led him to yet another level of insight, where he saw not only that the depth and growth of his farm existed for the purpose of providing food for the people nearby, but that it also had another purpose that he saw or more accurately felt when he looked into Kate's eyes, the fall of that bad storm.

Ivy Lily

During the summer, when Sun and Das taught classes at their home, there was a designated time that the students could ask questions. One day, everyone was silent and there were no questions. In response, Sun asked if anyone had a problem or a worry of some sort, and this got people talking. Small problems were raised: a broken down car, a sore muscle, etc. Then one lady from China, whose English wasn't proficient and who was quiet most of the time, began to speak about the small village she was from. A tsunami had hit her village. She had been trying to reach her family on the telephone for several days and each time the phone just kept ringing without any answer. As she spoke she became more and more upset, even hysterical, and Clara, who was listening, became concerned.

When the question-and-answer session ended, Clara looked for the lady from China. Her name was Ivy Lily, a double name. Clara asked her if she could be of help in some way. She then and there requested to be Clara's student. Clara was not taking new students at the time, especially students who were coming from overseas, as the work load was too great to complete in the short period of time that students who were coming from afar usually had allotted to themselves. But none of that mattered at the moment that Ivy Lily was requesting to be Clara's student. Clara accepted and over the course of the following year, Ivy Lily would travel to America to study with her.

Clara found out over time that Ivy Lily's father was a street sweeper in the village where she grew up. He woke at four every morning and by 4:30 he was sweeping. By nine AM he was finished. When he got home, he would sweep the family's house, which was large because Ivy Lily's father had four brothers who all had families living in this one house. Ivy Lily said that no one else in the house ever swept except her father, which was OK with him because he liked sweeping. He came up with stories while he swept, so the sweeping served as a catalyst for the dawning of these tales, later to be written down and read by Ivy Lily. He said that without the sweeping there would be no stories.

When Ivy Lily was in America, she stayed with her boyfriend Adam, who lived on the outskirts of Brooklyn in an area where many people originally from East Asia lived. It was quiet and more residential and less expensive than Manhattan. They lived simply in an apartment. Adam liked to meditate. He liked Ivy Lily's cooking and she could get most of the ingredients she was used to cooking with in China in their neighborhood, because so many Asians lived there. Ivy Lily told Adam her father's stories in addition to what Clara taught her, so that Adam went many different places in his mind without having to leave the apartment. Without the busyness of people around him and with the quiet of his neighborhood he continued on a journey where he could stay within himself and diminish what to him was unreal and kindle and make known what was real. Over the years, it was evident to Clara that Adam was working on himself continuously. The efforts that he put forth to dispel in himself what he called darkness were made up of practices he had been given by his teacher in Japan. These practices involved putting his body into positions that appeared easy to one who didn't practice them but were actually very difficult. It was the small, subtle movements that made them difficult, like pointing the toes or keeping the heels together.

These subtle movements made a huge difference to the level of difficulty, and the only way these movements could be maintained was through concentration. To Adam, what became more and more interesting about these movements was that they were controlled by the mind and established in Adam the realization that if the mind was peaceful it could control matter. Though Adam's teacher, simply called *sensei*, taught these difficult positions, he carried the same message of all the great spiritual masters: to realize the spirit, one must not harm others.

Clara was impressed by the changes she saw in Adam. Each time she saw him, which was not often since he rarely left the apartment, he was more at ease than the time before. It was hard to recollect how he was when they first met, but she could recall that he seemed worried, negative, shut down, and ill at ease, even in his movements. Over time, she could no longer remember him like that. It was clear that he was on a path, and that he had for a long time worked effortfully but now was being carried without any effort at all.

Sun and Das

By the end of the summer, Sun and Das's garden was abundant with vegetables but also with flowers. They had learned that vegetables liked flowers and that if certain flowers were planted near certain vegetables they would both do well. This was also true of vegetables next to vegetables. Sun said that tomatoes liked carrots and carrots liked tomatoes, so it was good to plant them next to each other. Similarly, it was good from time to time to change what was planted where, so one wasn't always planting tomatoes in the same exact place year after year.

What bothered Sun and Das about their garden was the way in which it had been cultivated. It started when they had to turn the soil and remove the plants already there, called weeds. Weeds are plants that society considers unwanted or not useful or even not nice to look at in comparison to those that are cultivated, like roses, irises, or tulips. Weeds are thought of as bitter tasting or poisonous when in fact many of them are medicinal and not poisonous at all. But in order to create space for a garden, the weeds had to be pulled from the earth, which Sun regarded as a form of murder. On the other hand, there were many insects, dragonflies, bees, butterflies, and many birds of all different colors living in their cultivated garden, and this gave Sun a sense of the life and goodness at work in their garden. Meanwhile, as Sun and Das were planting their garden year after year, they were also learning about what was already in the forest behind their house that they could eat. More and more, they realized that the forest provided many wonderful foods, so they combined the vegetables from the garden with wild edibles.

Sun and Das thought about the deaths of small creatures of the earth as a result of turning the soil to create a garden. Similar thoughts ran through the minds of ancient peoples who recited and sung prayers apologizing for the insects killed in the chaffing of wheat and honoring the lives of the even tinier insects killed when the wheat was cut; and later the microbes killed when the wheat was turned to flour; and even at the level of the organisms killed when the flour and water were baked and turned into bread. Without the recitation of these prayers, it was believed that the quality of nourishment in the bread was reduced to nothing.

To try to live a life of non-harming while pulling weeds up from the earth affirmed, to Sun and Das, how difficult it was to live a life completely free of non-harming. Yet they were determined and curious to see how far they could go and to what extent they could commit to a nonviolent life. They vowed to hold up, hold back, release, refrain from, and/or act upon, so as to cause the least harm to others.

For those who've lived through a war or other horrific conditions, it might be difficult to conceive of the pulling of weeds as a form of violence. Perhaps that was why for a time the ideas of Sun and Das were unpopular. But as time passed, it became apparent that seeing a weed as a part of oneself was an intimate way of seeing a weed, and it was this intimacy that made it then impossible to want to cause harm. What was realized in the one who cared for the weed was that the connection to the weed was a connection that went far beyond.

Howard

One summer day, Howard, Clara's neighbor and Ling's husband, experienced a shortness of breath and pain in his shoulder that became aggravated when he did anything physical. Howard didn't exercise in the usual sense but he worked hard in the garden and he made carvings out of wood and stone. After several days of feeling lousy, he became concerned and went to see a doctor. The doctor ran a variety of tests that showed his heart was weak. Howard was big and strong and had never in his seventy years thought of himself as anything but big and strong; so this news scared him. He wondered what it meant to have a weak heart?

Howard considered himself healthy and as a result was unconcerned with what most people are concerned with when it comes to health. He smoked cigars, drank whiskey, and ate heavy food without exercising. He never thought he would feel his health was threatened until those few days when he had a shortness of breath and pain in his shoulder. He changed many of his ways according to the doctor's instructions. He stopped smoking cigars, drinking whiskey, and eating heavy foods, and went regularly for long walks. But as well as those types of changes and with his mortality on his mind, he looked at everything differently—such that at this time, when Clara told Howard that Sun and Das respected the life of weeds and did not like pulling them, he understood.

Emmet

After the lecture that Clara gave under candlelight at Emmet's house, his guests thanked her for her wise words. She was often thanked for her words, but often did not know where they came from. She made a decision as she stepped into his house on that summer night, to speak of things she knew to be true. What that was she could not be sure of beforehand, but in the moment that she made that decision and stepped into the room where she would be speaking, it would, she hoped, come through, as it often did. It was these words, when they came through, that people were thankful for.

Clara

There were times in Clara's life where someone, usually close, said something to her that was hurtful. It took time for her to recover from these words, and sometimes she couldn't completely recover. Clara knew that such words were often untruths and tried not to react with harmful words. She discovered that if she did have something unkind to say, it was best if she waited a day. By the next day, she was always grateful she hadn't said what she would have said had she not waited. Of course, Clara had said mean things that she had regretted, mostly while quarreling, and it was even harder to recover from *her* harsh words than the harsh words of others. She had even written nasty letters that would have been very destructive had she not decided at the last minute not to send them. Once, after leaving such a letter with the secretary of someone whom she was upset with, she called the next day hoping that it hadn't yet been delivered. It turned out that the letter was still sitting on the secretary's desk. She asked the secretary to tear it up and asked her to promise it would never be seen by the person she'd been so upset with or by anyone else. After such experiences Clara often thought about her death and what the last thing she would say or communicate would be. . . .

Vincent

Vincent, who was for three years in retreat, could not hurt anyone through words during that time because he was in silence. When Vincent came out of his silence, it wasn't so much the cruel or discouraging things that people said to one another that surprised him as much as the words of insignificance: conversations based on irritations, complaints, and gossip—whole conversations about much of nothing, made up of putting others down, empty chatting, noise.

Frances

Frances told stories about her life, like the ones in books that her son Theo read, which conveyed truths about the experience of existence: stories about young girls whose mothers had died, or whose parents had no money, so the girls were sent to live in a convent. Frances would describe the dormitories and bunk beds, the meals of boiled potatoes and cabbage, how there was never enough of it and that the girls went to bed hungry. By the time Frances was done with her story, the listener felt a truth different from the ordinary complaints or irritations of the day and felt nourished by her words.

Vincent

When he came out of retreat, Vincent would tell stories of his retreat. No one knew when he would tell them, as it was never planned. From time to time, spontaneously, he would start singing the truths he'd realized in the middle of the desert, usually in the middle of the night, in his meditation. These songs of Vincent's were made up of phrases with multiple meanings, the basis of each of which was truth.

Bennett

Clara had bees in her house: first only one, then a day later, three; then ten; and after a few weeks, too many to count. She called her neighbors and they came over with a large jar, with a lid that had holes in it. They said that if you put beer in the jar, the bees would be attracted to the smell and fly in. But since there were so many bees, chances were that the bees had built a hive somewhere in the walls of the house that would have to be removed.

Clara called someone from the Yellow Pages who knew how to remove bees and their hives from homes. That was why Bennett and his assistant came and drove their truck through the field, past the roses, right up to the front door of the house. Bennett was an elderly man with a limp and hair dyed jet black, which looked strange on account of his having the face of an old man. He had bad psoriasis, especially on his elbows, was soft-spoken, and looked as if he spent a lot of time crying, because his eyes were wet and puffy. He had an accent, which Clara could not place, except that it told her he was not from the local area. His assistant was a much younger man who could have been his son, even though he called Bennett by his first name. It seemed that he looked up to and aimed to please the older man.

In no time at all, the beehive was located. The assistant went to get the ladder, which Bennett climbed up. The hive had to be removed and the bees flew around in a fury. Clara was afraid to get stung. While Bennett was on the ladder removing the hive, his assistant had located a praying mantis on a blade of grass near the house, which he carefully picked up and carried away from the house and into the woods. When Clara asked him what he was doing, he explained that the mantis would be safer in the woods than close to the house.

Eli

When Clara's father Eli was ten, he and his family lost their home in Vienna, which was at that time considered one of the most cosmopolitan cities in Europe. In the 1930s, anyone Jewish or of Jewish ancestry who owned property was no longer allowed any legal rights to their homes and businesses, and all the properties were claimed by the government. If any family argued for the ownership of their home, they were killed. The only thing they could do was leave their homes quickly, and go as far away as possible in the hopes they could again find a home somewhere else. Decades later, the government of Austria apologized for having stolen the homes of so many families. To support their apology, they conducted a search for any existing members of these families in the various places they had escaped to. The properties were offered back to the family members, and in the event that the family no longer wanted the property, money was offered. Eli and his cousin Marvin were notified and provided with such an "apology."

Eli fantasized about returning to Europe and living in his childhood house, while all along knowing that that was not, for numerous practical and emotional reasons, a real possibility. He therefore took the money offered and put it in a bank in Vienna. He rarely withdrew money from the account, except when he and Sarah were, on few occasions, on vacation in Europe. During the 1980s and 90s the interest rates were high, especially in Europe and the amount of money in the account grew. Marvin, on the other hand, did not fantasize about going back to Europe, nor did he want his portion of the money. Because the money was connected to the killings of so many, Marvin considered accepting it a form of stealing.

The story around the money was so painful that the two remaining relatives could never discuss it without it becoming a terrible argument. The different ways that the cousins reacted to the money could never be reconciled and caused a riff of tension between them that only grew stronger as time passed. It was not that Eli was without ideals that he took the money; it was just that his ideals were different from Marvin's. Marvin thought it important to trace the money back to its original purpose, which he saw as a formal apology for that which could never be forgiven, such that in some way had he taken any of the money, even a small amount, he would have felt linked to the crimes that the money was compensation for. Eli felt the Austrian government's efforts to track down the survivors and offer monetary rewards was an act of kindness. To Eli, the better way to respond to unkindness was through kindness and thus it was necessary to take the money in order to acknowledge the kindness, small as it might seem in comparison to all that was lost. In this way, though his childhood home, having been mortgaged and paid for by his father, was stolen just before the war years, Eli did not feel that he was stealing when he accepted the reparation money offered decades later.

When Eli died Sarah thought it best to take the money out of the account in Vienna and put it in a local bank in upstate New York. She did not have any sentimental or nostalgic feelings and ties toward Europe, like Eli had, which was for the greater part the reason why he'd left the money in Austria in the first place. However, Sarah rather than close the account over the phone did want to go to Vienna and meet with the banker, whose father had been a friend of Eli's, and whose grandfather had known Eli's father. Because Sarah was elderly and hadn't traveled in more than ten years—years during which Eli was hunched over in a chair complaining of chest pain and neither wanting to go anywhere nor be left alone at home—Clara accompanied her mother on the trip.

Clara and Sarah discovered that, without Eli ever letting on (for he never said how much money there was), Eli had a large sum of money by almost anyone's standards. Eli in his holey sweater, who lived on crackers and oranges, who never took taxis or stayed in nice hotels, who bought his fruit on the roadside but had paid for both of his children to go to college, was a rich man. This pained and delighted but most of all surprised Clara and Sarah. They spent a week in that most wonderful city, in a most wonderful hotel, happily spending Eli's money.

Sarah bought a vest with many pockets, pockets to keep money in, and found that after not having gone shopping in many years she liked smaller, high-end shops more than department stores. She bought some new underwear and took Clara to the opera. They went to the best bakery in the center of town and bought bread. Clara went to a frame shop— the same shop that apparently the emperor had bought gold frames for his family pictures more than two centuries previously. She bought wine glasses from the Art Deco period, hand-painted with flowers and birds. They were superbly packaged, so as not to break on her voyage back home, by the owners of the shop—two elderly sisters, elegantly dressed. Clara also bought a winter coat that came from Italy: black, with many zippers and drawstrings, and asymmetrical with a zigzag hem.

Considering the amount of money they now understood they had, Clara and Sarah didn't buy much. But compared to what they ordinarily would have purchased, they bought a lot. Years later, Clara thought they should have bought more but Sarah didn't have such thoughts. The problem was that Sarah felt a lot like Marvin did, so that by the end of their week in Vienna, Sarah felt heavy from her purchases and considered them frivolous. The feel of the money in her pockets, purse, and hands brought the unfathomable background to the foreground, so that it was a kind of stealing from those who'd lost their lives.

Clara didn't consider her and her mother's shopping spree to be a form of stealing, in the usual sense, any more than much of everything is stolen. Clara thought that the gold that decorated and plated the frames that she bought was stolen from the earth; the cotton of her new stylish coat was stolen from the cotton plant; and the cow's milk that anyone drank, outside of the cow's calf, was stolen from the cow. She thought wasting food, taking more than one needed or eating inattentively was stealing, when living in the city all she had to do was step outside her door to find a dog or a person who was hungry. She thought that everything that people thought they owned because they paid money for or inherited was really a loan, including the physical body. She thought that life in and of itself was so precious and valuable that just by being born one owed a huge debt, and that unless one lived in a spirit of service, free of feelings of entitlement, one was, if only perhaps in small ways, a thief.

Amala

Clara had a music teacher in India named Amala. Amala taught many things: dance, painting, herbs, but most often the Sanskrit language. She was a scholar and lover of grammar, and taught through singing. The tenses (past, present, and future), cases (nominative, vocative, accusative, instrumental, dative, ablative, genitive, and locative), pronouns (he, she, it, them, we, they, etc.), and the conjugations of verbs—all were put to melodies as a way to learn and memorize them. There were songs for masculine and feminine nouns or nouns that ended in vowels. There were songs that taught the eight cases of grammar through the telling of a story, and one story in particular Clara learned was about stealing.

The story was about a boy who gave a flower to a girl in the hopes that she would think he was great. At the time, he thought of the flower as his. The girl thought he was arrogant for thinking that. She said that the flower belonged to the earth and what was temporarily his was the act of offering it, but not the flower itself. Of course, the boy then fell in love with the girl and the singer of the song learns more than grammar. Clara liked this song a lot and so did Amala, for as Amala became a popular teacher and traveled the world, everywhere she went she taught this song. Thus, this song about the boy, the flower, and the girl, once known by only a few people in a small village, spread and was being sung in many places. Clara, having learned this song from Amala, taught it to Gazelle, Madeleine, and Ivy Lily; and Ivy Lily taught it to Adam; and when Ivy Lily went back to China, she taught it there, so that years later when Clara visited her, people knew this song. In this way, the knowledge of this song spread, as if carried by birds from the north to the south in winter.

Madeleine

It came to be that twelve years after Madeleine and Moses met, they had twins—a girl they named Emily and a boy named Elliot. The birth of the twins was celebrated by many. Though Madeleine had had some small difficulty at first getting pregnant, once she was, the pregnancy and the birth went smoothly. During the time that Madeleine was pregnant, she had a lot of energy to work on many projects and found that time to be exceedingly productive. She painted, gardened, baked cakes, wrote songs, recorded and produced albums, helped Moses with his documentary film, and assisted her friend Clara, who was writing a book of short stories. Her creative energy was at a high.

Madeleine had always been interested in the ways plants and animals as well as people reproduced, but while she was pregnant this interest increased and took on an emotional quality. At the grocery, she would pause in the dairy section and wonder about the animal whose eggs and milk had ended up in a carton. She thought about her own eggs and milk and how it was part of this birth-giving cycle that was enabling her and Moses to have children. During her pregnancy, Clara came to visit. She brought photos she had taken of the field behind her house. Years before, it had been a field of cut grass, but Clara had let it grow wild and flowers of all sorts filled the field. At first, there were only a few flowers, but the wind and birds had come and spread the seeds so that eventually the whole field was filled with flowers. Clara was grateful to have a house within such a field. When she explained to Madeleine how at first only a few flowers were there and what it had grown into, Madeleine thought of the reproductive systems in nature, in particular in flowers.

Madeleine told Clara a story about a whale that was 14,000 pounds and put in a tank so that people could come and see her. This was a way of making large sums of money, because the people who came to see her paid an entrance fee. Madeleine compared the size of the tank to the whale's original home of the ocean as minuscule. She said it would be like living in a space the size of a human fingernail.

Through artificial means, this mammal had been impregnated. When the baby whale was born, in no time at all the baby was taken and sent to another place far away where there was another tank with an entrance fee. For this had become a business, and for reasons that Clara and Madeleine could not understand many people came and paid the fee without—it seemed—thinking that sea creatures belonged in the ocean. When the baby whale was taken, the mother made a sound that none of the workers at the world of sea cages had heard before. This sound was recorded and researched by scientists who said it was a sound capable of traveling further than the far ends of the ocean. Such was the depth of the cry of the mother for her baby.

During Madeleine's pregnancy, she discovered a newfound reverence for reproductive cycles and was saddened by man's manipulation of it, especially when it came to animals. She didn't understand why her brother went fishing every year for his birthday. To keep the peace with her brother, she didn't confront him about his fishing trips, but she did teach to those who accepted her as a teacher another way of relating to animals, one that didn't involve hooking, caging, killing, or eating them.

Emily and Elliot were raised similarly to Barry and Bethel, the children of Solon and Esther, Clara's brother and his wife, in that they were not given things in order to get them to behave a certain way. They were given things, but not as rewards; and sometimes they weren't given things for a variety of reasons, but not as a punishment. The main emphasis in both households was not placed on things and the children in their requests were actually, naturally, quite reasonable. This, it seemed, contributed to Barry and Bethel living simply when they became adults. Also, since Esther worked with a population of people who were financially poor, her children had grown up seeing their mother give most of her things away. In this manner, they were not afraid to go without or with less. They did not live in excess, nor had they as children. Small gifts at times were given and emphasis was placed on the quality in which they were given and received.

Clara

An estranged cousin of Clara's married a wealthy man, the son of one of the most powerful lawyers in Boston. The endless varieties and enormous quantities of food served at the wedding upset Clara. The desire to serve a meal to the guests who had traveled a distance to celebrate the couple's love, she understood. Offering food and nourishment as part of love and life, she understood. But when it is taken beyond a reasonable amount of food for a festive meal, the reason for the celebration gets lost. Such were the thoughts of Clara and as it turned out also of Esther at the wedding. Both of them had looked into the eyes of a hungry being, child, adult, or animal, and those were the memories that surfaced that night at the wedding, such that they felt embarrassed for the wedding couple.

Wise One

Wise One traveled from time to time across the world to teach his students. Arun offered and took on the responsibility of organizing his trips. This was complicated as Wise One traveled with his entire family. Arun put together a schedule for Wise One that included first and foremost teaching but also left room for sightseeing and spending time with students. Clara invited Wise One and his family to her home and he accepted.

Wise One had never been to Clara's home. From the time she knew he was coming to the time he was to arrive, she had one week to get things ready. Clara spent the week cleaning. There was nothing she did not clean. She washed the ceilings, floors, and walls, all the windows and their sills. She washed the refrigerator inside and out, and the glass on all the framed pictures. She went through and organized every drawer and folded all of her and Theo's clothes nicely. She cleaned under, on top, and inside of things until everything was clean. She did not want dust on the pictures, windows, mirrors, floors, walls, or under the day bed. She did not want the water that the flowers were in, the bed sheets, or the teakettle to be dirty. She loved her home, she loved Wise One, and she loved cleaning. Therefore, cleaning her home in honor of Wise One's visit made her happy. Clara had, like most people, experienced some close calls in her life. She had experienced enough pain and suffering that she was happy having a home with things in it to clean, and a teacher, or loved one, willing to come visit.

On the day that Wise One was expected, he telephoned to say he would not be coming. Clara received this news with complete equanimity. She was not attached to the outcome of her cleaning and cooking because the cleaning and cooking themselves had brought her much joy. Through cleaning her home, it was as if she had scrubbed her body and mind, and she herself felt clean. She thought of the ways in which one could welcome another and saw the act of cleaning as a valuable one. A cat, when given the choice, will sleep in a clean spot over a dirty one. In fact, animals, when they are dying, will continue to groom themselves, such that when they die, they die clean. After Eli died, Sarah stopped cleaning. But by the time Sarah had worked through her grief, or most of it, or what she could possibly work through, the first sign of coming out of that grief was that she started cleaning again.

Clara thought back on her visit with Lucy to the monastery, far off in time and location. The monks' quarters were always clean. This made it easier for them to study and pray. Frances, at the age of ninety-four and still living by herself, would keep her body and apartment clean one section at a time. When she was old and fragile, Mother Teresa would help anyone in need of keeping themselves or their surroundings clean by going to their house and cleaning. She often found the insides of houses of those who were elderly, lonely, or sick to be neglected, and part of her service (which she always said was for Jesus) was cleaning.

Clara

Clara was departing from a wonderful visit with Madeline and Moses, and while waiting to board the plane, she looked around at the people in the airport and wondered how many of them were content. For the most part, she thought they looked unhealthy and stressed or pressed for time. Perhaps the airport isn't the best place to ask oneself such questions or to make such generalizations. Clara thought about her own life, whether or not she was content, and if so, where that contentment had come from. She felt content when one or both of her cats lay on her chest and purred. Gazelle was content because in the various neighborhoods where she lived after she turned nineteen bombs weren't exploding. She thought most of the people around her who were discontent were spoiled. Emmet was content, blind. Ivy Lily was content commuting an hour in each direction to study with Clara. Adam was content sitting on his meditation cushion and rarely leaving the apartment.

When Kate and her husband lost their fall crop and half a year's income, they counted their blessings and thought many times over how things could have been worse. Clara was content when, after she broke all her bones and lay in bed for a year, for the first time since her accident she could walk to the end of the hallway and back. At that time, she thought that as long as she could walk she would be content; but Frances, at ninety-four and with walking abilities that were diminishing all the time, was still content. Meanwhile, others threw temper tantrums over a cup of coffee or having to wait for five or ten minutes or over a misunderstanding—something that was not even real. Clara thought about whom she knew was content or not, including herself, and it seemed to her that it was not entirely dependent on externals or circumstances; that it could be that someone with a lot of difficulties or challenges felt in essence satisfied, and that it was this essential satisfaction that gave one pleasure in the externals of one's life. Similarly, if one did not have this essential satisfaction, one's inner discontent could spoil everything.

Clara wondered whether Vincent during his three years of retreat was content, and what it was like for him to come out of his solitude. She imagined he would be content for the rest of his life and could teach others from where contentment came.

Clara was content when she was with Wise One. Now that he was no longer in his physical form, she could still be with him, but it was up to her to push herself in the way that Wise One just through his presence could get her to do. Clara worked hard on the practices that Wise One, Sun, and Das had given to her, incorporating movement with breath and systems of counting the number of breaths to the number of movements, bringing about rhythm and organization in the body and in life.

These practices purify the body, the vessel, but only if one works past levels of acquired strength. It was only when acquired strength was exhausted that one used one's innate strength and Clara's teachers had ways of getting people to work that hard. Out of that work one realized capabilities within oneself that otherwise would have gone unnoticed. This realization of their potential helped many to let go of feelings of inadequacy or incompetence, such that they became great teachers themselves, experienced in what was taught.

Madeleine

During the time that Madeleine was pregnant, Clara made several trips from her home in the mountains to Madeleine's house in one of the southern states, where everything was flat and mostly hot. Near Madeleine's house was a Hindu temple and it seemed that every time Clara visited it was a Hindu holiday, so there were a lot of festivities at the temple that both women enjoyed going to. On one occasion, the festival of Ganesh Chaturthi, at the end of the evening program a blessing was made and flowers were offered to everyone there. When it was Clara's turn to receive the flowers, the priest's helper, an elderly woman (a grandmother, perhaps even a great grandmother) put a few petals into her hand. The woman's touch was firm rather than gentle, and reassuring. When Clara opened up her hand, she saw that the flower petals had been cut many times so that what were in her hands were not flower petals but pieces of flower petals—tiny pieces of reds and yellows. Both Clara and Madeleine appreciated and were pleased by the tiny petal pieces. When the time came to offer the pieces back to the deity a few minutes later, everyone pushed forward as there was no hesitance in giving them back and prostrating to the deity. Clara and Madeleine went home feeling content and serene from their temple experience.

On another occasion, when Madeleine had gone to the temple, an eight-year-old boy sung a song for Krishna's birthday. The song was full of dissonant melodies, slightly off tune but even more beautiful because of it, and Madeleine was entranced by the song. Afterwards, Madeleine, thirty-five years old, asked the boy if he would teach it to her. He told her *no*, that it would be too difficult for her. She appreciated his answer but told him she was up for it, that she was a hard worker, and would apply herself and practice a lot. She said that she had learned other difficult songs and had been studying consistently for years. She was persuasive and he finally agreed to teach her.

Later, Madeleine met the boy's parents and they were impressed with her. They could tell her desire for learning was great. She had many lessons with the boy. She found time every day to practice and learned the song well. He told her that anyone singing this song regularly was protected by Krishna and Madeleine felt this to be true. Finding time to practice was easy for Madeleine. She could lay things out for herself well. She could push herself in ways that most could not unless they were being forced. She did not know at that time how much she would grow to love that boy.

Rupa and Vidya

When anyone came to the clinic located in the suburbs of Sarana, whether it was to live or work, Rupa and Vidya were happy. The show of warmth expressed was unique to the clinic and to them. Rupa always wore brightly colored skirts made up of traditional and local designs and Vidya always wore plain gray trousers and a short-sleeved button-down shirt. Once, when Clara was at the clinic, one of the children was calling out the multiplication tables—"eight times two is sixteen, eight times three is twenty-four, eight times four is thirty-two, and eight times five is forty," and just kept going and going. Rupa ran across the room and picked him up. She was so happy and proud.

The clinic was basically one room and the children who lived there were grateful for their situation. Clara remembered the first time she visited. She sat in the waiting room and even without talking to anyone felt cared for by the atmosphere alone. She noticed that the children who were more functional helped the others with more severe difficulties. The room had lots of windows and the air blew across the room pleasantly. Out of the windows you could see the coconut grove and, in it, the trees blowing with the wind. During monsoon season it would rain heavily every afternoon for ten minutes and the windows and doors would be closed. The laundry hanging on the line to dry was quickly brought in and then, when the rain stopped, taken out again.

Clara

Clara sat at her kitchen table having breakfast. While reading the newspaper, she stumbled on an obituary, and realized by the dates given that the deceased had been younger then she. Several close friends of hers had died relatively young of different cancers and one of her friends had a ten-year-old son with a rare form of kidney disease. The paper also brought news of war, flooding, famine, and different types of suffering that she herself was not experiencing.

Clara put down the paper and as she had woken early and had some extra time went back upstairs and slipped into bed, under the covers, for the cool morning air of fall had arrived. She propped herself up with two pillows, taking hers and Theo's (for Theo was long out of bed, waking up most mornings at an hour that almost everyone would consider the middle of the night), and opened up *Folly*, the novel she was reading by Susan Minot. Enjoying her free time, her novel, and lying in bed, she thought of the news in the paper and the obituaries. She looked out of the window at the trees whose leaves were changing color and already falling.

Later that day, Clara and Theo drove to Sarah's house for dinner and on the way the traffic was moving slowly on account of a bad accident. Three vehicles were smashed together and turned upside down. After passing the accident, they drove slower and more carefully than usual as did everyone else on the highway; the accident served as a reminder that life was precious and fleeting. When they got to Sarah's, she was surprised to see them, for though they had spoken with her that morning she had forgotten they were coming. One thing she never forgot was one of the houses she had lived in as a child in England during the war. It was an old stone house, built right up to the edge of the road. She said the woman of the house was emotionally intuitive and had wanted to adopt her younger brother, ten at the time, whom Sarah had not spoken to in years.

At the end of their evening at Sarah's, Theo and Clara hurried to the bus station so that Clara could catch the bus to New York City. When they arrived, it turned out that she had read the schedule incorrectly and the next bus wasn't due for another two hours. Clara was frustrated having to wait for a bus she had rushed for. She turned and spoke for a few minutes about her frustration to a lady sitting and waiting for the same bus. When she was finished, the lady who it seemed did not mind listening told Clara that the two hours that she would have to wait would pass. Clara thought, *yes, it will pass*, and that actually her whole life would pass. It seemed that in those few words the lady expressed an important truth. Clara said she was going across the street to the diner to get a cup of tea and asked the lady if she wanted some. The lady said, "No thank you." Then Clara suggested an herbal tea like mint, and it seemed like it might have been a very long time (if at all) since the lady had had a mint tea. The lady smiled and accepted it, saying that it would be nice. Clara went to the diner feeling happy to have met this lady and to be bringing her tea.

Vincent

Once, Clara went to visit Vincent while he was on retreat. He and a small group of other retreatants had requested of Lama Daniel to ask a visitor to come and give teachings and tell them things from the outside world that would help prepare them for their return when the retreat was over. This was a rare and brief period when the retreatants were allowed to see one another and have a teacher visit. Their retreat had a lot of structure: in certain periods they were each in isolation, unable to receive letters or even to read or write; at other times they could gather together, never to speak, but to meditate or sing with each other or share a meal. Some of them at times did read, write, study, or work on translating old sacred texts written in ancient languages. Some wrote music or poetry or painted pictures. On the occasion that Clara visited, each retreatant gave her a gift, a show of appreciation for her coming. These offerings were small, a pebble wrapped in string, homemade almond milk, a flower pressed between two pieces of paper. Clara drank the milk and put the offerings in her pocket. She felt a world of contentment behind them.

Madeleine and Moses

Emily and Elliott, Madeleine and Moses's children, were from an early age curious about where they had come from. When Madeleine spoke of times in her life when she was younger, the twins asked if they had been there. Madeleine would say *no*, that it was before they were born and they would wonder what it meant to be born. When the twins were four, Madeleine became pregnant again with what turned out to be a girl. As Madeleine's body was changing and she and Moses were preparing for the newborn, the twins had a lot of questions about themselves and their new brother or sister, especially how it happened and where he or she would come from. Madeleine answered these questions in ways she thought suitable for the child's mind. She compared the bird's nest in the tree to her belly and that she too had once been in the bird's nest of her own mother's belly. She also explained that to a certain extent where we come from was a mystery and that we could never know everything. She spoke of slow invisible processes and planting seeds and watching them grow. Moses on the other hand thought it was important to "tell it like it is." He talked of sex, desire, and attraction. The children were interested in what both parents had to say.

Emmet

Emmet, who did not have children and never married, wore a wedding ring. He said he was married to God. In that way, he was like a nun or a monk, although different from the monastics, as he was not celibate. He loved wearing his ring, which was a traditional wedding band, and it looked pleasing on his finger, like it belonged there. If he forgot to put it on, his hand looked bare, as if something was missing. He had decided that his way of being creative would be through his paintings. They were to him like his children, and he made many and they were loved by many and ended up in homes and museums throughout the world. The objects in them were old, forgotten, broken, thrown out, or no longer useful, yet in the pictures they were resurrected. Objects from previous times, faded from most people's memories, nonexistent to the younger generation, were made current again.

When Emmet was in the hospital, after his fall, he had two primary visitors—his mother and his girlfriend—one on each side of the bed. It had been hard for Emmet's mother to accept her son's girlfriend because she was from Jamaica and her skin couldn't have been darker or her accent, to Emmet's mother, more difficult to understand. But during those months, a once-antagonistic relationship between his mother and his girlfriend turned into one of love, especially as Emmet's mother saw that the woman from Jamaica loved Emmet no less because of his handicap and did not question her future with him. So, literally over Emmet's thin, long body, for he was almost too tall for his hospital bed and his hospital gown, through nights when Emmet could have easily slipped away from both of them, his mother accepted his girlfriend, and overcame the deep prejudice and narrow view-points that had informed her way of looking for most of her life.

Frances

Frances knew that she would die soon and looked back on her life, scrutinizing her actions: some good that she was proud of, and other actions limited by a lack of understanding that over time she came to understand, and was also proud of that understanding that came to her late in life. Each day, little by little, she went through her things, organizing, eliminating, letting go. She remembered times in her life when she had stood up for someone whom she felt was humiliated, demoralized, or insulted. She said the workers in this country were the real nobility, but that with the invention of the assembly line they had been driven crazy.

The things that remained of Frances's were of value to her and maybe would have value for her children. Her clothes were handmade and showed her combination of resourcefulness and creativity. Her collection of books—works by Kafka, Chekhov, Simone Weil, Tolstoy, the *Bhagavad Gita*—were all hardcover and, if not first editions, then editions from long ago. Inside the books along the margins were notes, written in pencil in

Italian and in cursive script. Whether these notes added or diminished the value of the books would vary, depending on what type of person was holding the book. Since none of her children nor their spouses could read Italian, since Theo lived in a small cabin and enjoyed using the public library, and since Theo's sister lived in a small crowded apartment on a six-floor walk up with her husband and their child, Frances wondered what would happen to her books and assumed her children would not want them.

Adam

Adam had a routine, which included meditating three times a day. Ivy Lily joined him in the evenings at the end of a long day, but eventually sat with him in the morning, too. Over time, she learned many things about meditation. When asked to talk about what she had learned, not knowing English well and having a poetic nature her descriptions were metaphoric. One she frequently used was of water—whether it was still, moving, turbulent, in drops like rain, or in large masses like lakes and oceans. She used her hands and arms to help in her explanations.

She explained that the mind was by nature transparent, such that the light of intelligence could emit its rays through the mind. But when the mind was cloudy, this light was covered and this caused many problems. She said the mind was like a glass of water and if you put a few drops of yellow coloring and then red, blue, and green, and kept adding colors, you would end up with black water you couldn't see through. She compared the spectrum of colors to the thoughts of the mind, and defined meditation as colorless water. She said the mind of someone who meditated a lot could understand things easily. She said that such a person was unafraid of the body's deterioration, decay, and disgusting nature, because she or he understood that it was impermanent and could see what was lasting underneath, because of their clear mind.

Perhaps this was why Theo could spend so much time at work cleaning people of blood and feces. Sometimes he would clean a patient and change the bedding and have to do it all over again an hour later. He never confused the physical body with the soul he was taking care of.

Theo

Theo's work at the hospital was demanding even on a "good" day, which he had more often than not once he stopped working in a big city hospital. Smaller hospitals outside of cities weren't as under-resourced as one might think. Theo found nurses who were very caring, whom he could look up to and learn from, and he was more excited about his profession than he had been in a long time. But one day he almost quit, as the work pushed beyond even Theo's threshold.

Theo had a patient who was diabetic and had gangrene in one of his legs. It was spreading quickly and the only way to stop it was to remove the leg. The leg was amputated and immediately afterwards it was Theo's job to keep the wound clean and freshly bandaged. This had to be done every hour. As is usually the case, the patient was upset, demoralized, and afraid, as was the patient's family.

The wound was extreme and the cleaning had to be done slowly because it demands care. But it also had to be done quickly because the patient experiences even more pain when the wound is touched. Having cleaned the wound already several times that day, Theo came to do a mid-day cleaning. The wound had turned a strange green color, a rotten odor filled the room, and the patient and his wife were crying. Theo was tired, his feet hurt, and he hadn't had time for lunch. He stepped out of the room looking for another nurse or doctor to help him, but everyone was as busy as Theo and there was no nurse's aid around. So he went back into the room. He looked down at the wound and thought about quitting his job, walking out—away from the stench, the wound, and the look of fear in his patient—and going to the park, where the air was fresh and people were relaxed. There he would eat his lunch.

He thought about the work ahead of him, cleaning the wound, washing it carefully to make sure it didn't get infected and/or even worse. He thought that even if he cleaned the wound now, in another hour he would have to do it all over again. For one moment he stood there and thought to himself, *This is it. I can't take it any longer. I can't do this work anymore. It's too hard. I've reached my limit.* Then after a pause, he realized the wound needed cleaning and that he was there to do it. The bandage was already in his hands. The family was depending on him. There was no extra nurse floating around the floor that he worked on. So he pulled himself together, did an especially good job, and found out qualities about himself he never knew he had.

Iris

When Clara was forty, she inherited a camera. The camera was roughly a hundred years old, made out of wood, with a German lens. It was a large-format camera, which meant it took one piece of film at a time. Each piece of film was five by seven inches and slid into a holder that itself slid into the back of the camera, called the "camera back." The camera was completely manual: nothing was automatic, electric, battery-operated, or digital. Though it seemed simple enough—a box with a tiny hole on one side and a piece of film on the other so that light traveled through the hole and box and left impressions of the external world on the film—Clara could not figure out how to use it. So she called Louise, one of her dearest friends, who knew someone named Iris, whom she thought could help Clara, if Clara paid her. Clara had some savings and could afford to have someone help her, so she telephoned Iris, and a few days later Iris came.

Iris was a young woman, half Clara's age, who had recently graduated from college. Her major was photography and she'd just spent the last four years either taking pictures or in the dark room developing them. She had long brown hair that she wore in a twist that was always falling off the top of her head to one side or another. Her wardrobe came from thrift shops; she never bought anything new, had her own style, and always looked spiffy. Right away they liked each other. Clara told her that she liked the name Iris because it was the name of a purple flower that she loved. Iris told her that she liked it, too, but more because the iris was the part of the eye used for seeing. Funnily enough, Clara had not thought of this. When she thought of the name Iris, it was Iris Murdoch who came to mind. Iris Murdoch had said that education was important not because it made someone happy but rather because it refined one's mind such that one could perceive happiness.

When Clara handed Iris the camera it was still in its case, and Clara found even the case hard to open. Iris questioned whether originally there might have been a key for the case but eventually prized it open by using a bobby pin that she took from her hair. Once it was out of its case, Iris took the whole camera apart in order to figure out its mechanics. Clara was wondering if Iris would be able to put the camera back together and Iris answered with an honest, "Probably." By the time Iris had taken the camera apart and put it back together, several hours had passed. Clara knew that Iris had a lot to teach her, and asked her if she could return.

Iris lived with her boyfriend Simon in an old rented house in a small town near Clara. The house was on a busy road, but to make up for that they had a large back yard with high grasses and many trees, where there was a good amount of wildlife, especially in the warmer months when Iris would tell Clara about all the different birds that she had seen in her yard: blue jays, cardinals, robins, crows, hummingbirds, ducks, sparrows, and occasionally a lone gray heron. Simon was a baker and a cyclist. He baked mostly bread and went for long bike trips, cycling sometimes for days. In his baking he experimented a lot and was always improving on some kind of sourdough rye, lemon poppy spelt, or eight-grain. Eventually, after at first doing most of his baking in the small kitchen in their house and then later in a bigger kitchen that belonged to the church, Simon built a wood-burning oven made from bricks in their back yard where he could bake many loaves of bread at once.

Iris was devoted to Simon; she admired him greatly, enjoyed living with him, and would have done anything for him. This was a quality that she had most especially for Simon, but Iris had a lot of devotion in general. She believed in others, their capacities and goodness, and wanted to be of service in any way possible. When Simon ultimately won prizes for both his long- and fast-cycling abilities and the tastes and textures of his bread, he knew that it was Iris who'd seen his gifts and encouraged him.

This was true in Iris's relationship to Clara as well, because Iris believed in Clara's vision of the world through her old and large camera. The belief that Iris had in Clara's artistry enabled her to help Clara more than anyone had ever done before, so that Clara's pictures within a few years of working with Iris became compelling. Though Iris herself was a photographer, she wasn't jealous or insecure in a way that might have prevented her from assisting Clara so generously. Iris did not in any way hold back her creativity or knowledge. If she could make a picture of Clara's better, she did.

Ani Chunzom

Every year, Clara spent a long weekend at a retreat center on the other side of the river, where the land was less mountainous than where she lived, but equally rural. That area had a lot of farms on winding country roads, where the houses were quite far from one another. The retreat center was an old hotel and many great teachers came through to lead retreats or give teachings, including Sun and Das. Once a year, Clara treated herself to a weekend with a Buddhist nun named Ani Chunzom. Ani Chunzom had long ago been married and later divorced. Because she became a nun at the age of fifty and had borne children and been an elementary school teacher, she knew a lot about family life, which enhanced her ability to relate to her students and they to her, since for the most part they weren't nuns and had families. Ani Chunzom's husband had had an affair and the divorce was painful with a lot of heated and negative emotions. The divorce actually led her to Buddhism, where through the grace of her teachers she was able to go deeply into practices of meditation and discover a way within herself to forgive her husband. As time passed, she became a powerful teacher.

The practices that Ani Chunzom taught were connected to those the avatars have taught, and these practices were thousands of years old.

All along, people have needed practices to keep their minds from being disturbed. At these retreats, the levels of practitioners were varied: some hadn't ever meditated; others had been meditating for decades. At the beginning of these retreats, it was common for Ani Chunzom to lead a partner exercise where for a period of four minutes two people came together—one as speaker, the other as listener. They told the other how they were feeling and when the time was up switched places or roles and the talker became the listener. There was something about the atmosphere around Ani Chunzom that people felt safe in and a lot was disclosed in these exchanges. Clara realized and was reminded of how much pain and suffering are in people's lives. It seemed that over the years of attending these retreats she had never had a partner who was happy. Divorce, betrayal, financial worries, career disappointments, illness, agitation, shyness, inability to sleep, chronic fatigue, poor eating habits, a sick child, time in prison, lack of discipline . . . pain and suffering spoken of by the ones with pain and suffering. This affirmed again in Clara's mind the need for guidance, pathways and practices, teachers, books and time: time to practice, reflect, and live well, so that one could get out of this suffering.

Theo

After thirty years of practice and study, Theo was knowledgeable in Tai Chi. Clara had learned a little of what's called "the form" from Theo. The form was made up of movements and each movement had a name. The names were in Chinese but had been translated into other languages and she knew some of these names: picking the needle from the haystack, picking the needle from the ocean floor or the sea bottom, fair lady weaving left side, fair lady weaving right side, playing the fiddle, waving clouds, or cross hands. She thought of these names and their corresponding movements strung together to make a form, and felt they held clues to ways where one could suffer less and be happy. She knew that to pick a needle from a haystack would require effort, but also knew that what took effort would become effortless over time. Clara loved watching Theo practice his form. It was soft, quiet, fluid, and graceful, and behind it there was a reservoir of energy and power.

Venerable K.

Clara had a friend named Venerable K., who was a devotee of Lama Daniel and in the same small group of retreatants as Vincent. On the rare occasions they could have visitors, twice a year for three years, Clara saw them both. Vincent was in a cabin far off, and Venerable K. was also in a cabin, but on the other side of the mountain from Vincent and the others, and saw no other structures where people were living for miles. From Venerable K.'s side of the mountain, all one could see was mountains. It was quiet there, so quiet that when Clara walked on the dried grass she made an effort to step lightly so as not to make noise, except during snake season, when she walked with a long stick, tapping it on the ground a few feet ahead of her to let the snakes know she was approaching. She was afraid of snakes, bees, scorpions, bears, foxes, tarantulas, and animals in general. She loved them but feared them simultaneously, and because of this strongly admired Venerable K. for living with the animals and feeding them directly from her hand.

Venerable K. had a caretaker, someone who came twice a month with provisions from the nearest city, four hours away. The food was left in a box in a wagon, just outside the Venerable's gate. She carried the box inside, put things away in her refrigerator or in closed jars so as not to attract animals, and returned the empty box to the wagon. Later, the caretaker would come and get the box and the wagon. It was all done in such a way that over the three years they never saw each other. Venerable K. got used to eating foods in the order of how quickly they would perish: fruits first, vegetables second, bread third, grains fourth, etc. and Clara thought that when Venerable K. finished her retreat and all foods at any time would be available to her, she would miss this system of eating.

Venerable K. had a lot of gratitude for her provisions, the perishables like kale and oranges, and the longer-lasting foods, like rice and beans.

She also had gratitude for her caretaker and all the people from whom the caretaker had gathered funds, not only for her food and other supplies but also for the building of her hut made from straw bales and heated by solar energy. This gratitude for food and water and those who brought it existed on a gross and subtle level. When Clara had the chance to eat food that Venerable K. prepared, while in retreat but also afterwards, the food tasted of this thankfulness and appreciation.

The retreatants lived in an area called a *tsam*, which had been created during a ceremony of prayers where a certain amount of distance from a designated center is measured in arms' lengths, by walking away from the center to the periphery. This circle serves as an area that protects the meditators from distraction while separating them physically from the rest of the world. The retreatants are expected to remain in the *tsam* for the duration of their retreat. When Clara was in the *tsam* the group of meditators she saw, immersed in their silence, were prepared for the strong winds and shielded from the sun and rain by hats and umbrellas. With these simple coverings from the elements of the terrain where they had settled to live without leaving for more than three years, they were content to the extent that the ordinary endless unhappiness of being thrown by the ups and downs of life without a stable feeling underneath was no longer a reality.

The mistaken perception of ebb, flow, and change as one's true nature was surrendered. Through their silence, they had established neutrality. Their meditations, quietude, grateful ways of eating, and the equanimity that resulted were the fruits of the preparations made over years of spiritual practices and disciplines taken by Venerable K. and Vincent and their group of close friends, who made their way into the vast lands forgotten by many, situated on the borders of this country. When the retreat was finished, the thread, ribbon, and rope that marked the circle of the *tsam* would be cut and the goodness and merit accumulated inside would spread to where it was needed.

Clara knew that when she returned home to Theo it would be cold and dark. It would be winter. He would have a fire going in the wood stove and perhaps some small sadness alongside of the fire for Clara having been gone, yet again, and for having to be the one to always make the fire to keep himself and the cats warm. She did not want to react to the entry into a new season with dread, for the winter was for many not the favorite of seasons. But Clara did not mind it because she liked wearing layers of clothes, sleeping with blankets one on top of another, and eating cooked foods.

Frances

While Clara had been traveling in the desert, Frances had been sick. Being sick was hard for Frances because in her ninety-one years she had experienced almost no sickness outside of the tuberculosis that she and everyone around her in the 1930s and 40s had had (along with hunger, war, and poverty), which left her, at nineteen, almost on her death bed. However, after that time, for the rest of her life she was healthy, strong, and stubborn, until this most recent bout of the flu, as winter approached.

During this time that she had the flu, the philosophies that she held dear, studied, and reflected upon for decades held her effortlessly in a calm, so that she no longer complained of all that she had complained of: the inefficacy of her exercises, the difficulty getting her mail, her lack of appetite, the fact that nothing good was ever on TV, etc. She wasn't worried about her money or the cost of things and she had no fear of death. She didn't want to be pressured about anything. She would answer the door or the phone, eat or bathe only if she felt like it, and in this way she was peaceful. If you were in her apartment fussing over her, explaining to her that her exercises were actually working, wrapping her in sweaters against the cold, or setting up the window fan if it was hot, she would let you do these things, not at all for her sake but because she saw that it made her visitor happy to feel useful.

Like this, time passed and Frances was still alive at the age of a hundred, breathing slowly and quietly, but breathing, and pausing when she wanted, in between the flow of breath, to feel the force of life still in her. This exchange with the world, of its air going in and out, was the ultimate ritual for which she was grateful.

At the end of her life, she spent most of her time lying in bed breathing, conscious of the inhale and exhale. Breathing in and out was as complete a cycle as the four seasons of the year or the twenty-four hours of a day. She could feel the subtle places where the breath reached both in and around her and knew that something, not nothing, was there. This sensation of the breath, especially when she was lying on her back, was sometimes enough for her to feel a current, where her mind and body was still and at the center of it all was a deep sense of wellbeing.

She had no words to describe this experience, so she'd just say that she wasn't going to say anything. Even if she didn't say anything, if she was lying on her back aware of the in- and outgoings of her breath, its movements and pauses, and you were in her room or in the apartment somewhere nearby, then you were in an atmosphere of beauty without any coverings or concealments or even objects, and so it was a blessing to be with Frances.

During those times, there was no longer anything for her to offer such as the meals she had once made of polenta, dandelion greens, and sautéed mushrooms; or the sewing and repairing of her children's clothes; or the long philosophical, spiritual, and political conversations; or her viewpoints. Yet without offerings there were offerings: they were nuanced, atmospheric, subtle, soft, and un-concrete. In the lucidity of her mind—lucid from observing the movements of her breath—she was leaving the material world behind for another phenomenon . . . like the Buddha's teaching about the raft that one needs to cross the ocean and no longer needs when one has reached the shore.

BOOK III: Ash

Adam

One day when Adam was on the platform in Coney Island waiting for the New York City subway train, he saw a woman leave a kitten on a bench and walk away. It was an odd time of day for travel in the city, for Adam worked unusual hours and there weren't many people around. No one else witnessed this act of abandonment. Adam, who'd never had a cat or any other animal to care for, could not help but go to the kitten. The kitten was small enough to fit in the palm of his hand. Once the kitten was in his hand he could not put the kitten back on the bench without feeling that he then would be adding to the act of abandonment. So he put the kitten in his coat pocket, and when his train to Manhattan arrived, got in.

Still holding the kitten in his pocket, he felt her licking his hand. He decided to keep the kitten and call her Wei, Chinese for great strength, for the kitten had awoken in him a compassion that he'd never experienced before. This was years before Ivy Lily came to live with Adam; but when Ivy Lily did come she said that she had seen Wei in her dreams and that Wei was a Buddha in a cat form. So it was that Adam reflected on the day the kitten was left on the bench, as if she had been God testing him, and that somehow the reward for his passing the test was Ivy Lily, who was sweet and pretty and had had visions of the cat. So Adam, Ivy Lily, and Wei came to live together and were able to live harmoniously in the held space of their minds and the simple two-room apartment in Coney Island.

The love between Adam, Ivy Lily, and Wei grew as they learned more about one another. They enjoyed each other's company in the home they set up. Adam was good at cleaning and taking care of plants and Ivy Lily purchased several original ink drawings of the Buddha and hung them on the walls in the apartment. Adam had an altar and on it were offerings to the Buddha of water, fruits, and flowers. Ivy Lily placed a picture of her parents on the altar, some incense, and rice from her country. Lighting candles and sitting at the altar, making these offerings, created a conducive space to meditate in.

When Clara came to visit and walked into their home she understood why Adam chose to stay at home as much as he did. Once, when Clara was traveling from north to south India and on the train for many days, stopping at every local stop and often remaining there for hours, she was content and did not feel the need to get off the train, go, or arrive anywhere. It had been so rare for her to be somewhere and not want to be somewhere else, and with the absence of that restlessness came a feeling of completion.

While it wasn't India passing by with the viewpoint of a train traveler, the life of Adam passed through the window of his mind, and he let it pass, while sitting on his meditation cushion, always feeling that although he didn't physically go anywhere, he was on a journey where he was in stillness, moving toward a place he wanted to go or rather return to. In this way, the current that Adam swam in, which for so long was one he felt he had to swim against, was now carrying him like a stream, without any effort of his own in a stretch that was unbroken, in time that was passing, without any grip on him. During these periods, the phone never rang, or at least he never heard it, so it never disturbed him.

Frances

When Frances was ninety-five she no longer left her apartment. She lived on a busy street but because the windows did not face the street, she herself often said, "You wouldn't know I live in New York City." Though she had loved New York (like a lot of immigrants who came from Europe around the time of the war), she also loved not knowing that she was in New York, especially since the New York that she'd lived in and experienced for the most part was no longer there. Frances said, "Now I live inside the door. My life outside the door is over, but that's OK." Frances had outlived all of her friends and family outside of her children, but said they were present inside the door. "Frank, Birdie, Marananta, Joseph, Yelena, Virginia, Tony: they are all here." In her mind she was among many.

Frances knew that if she told the social worker and physical therapist who occasionally came by (not because she wanted them to, but because Theo and his sister insisted) that her family and friends were all there living with her, because of the fact that she lived alone they would think she was "cuckoo." But, she said, "I am not cuckoo. I bathe and dress myself, do the dishes, make the bed, read Dante, and sew the holes in my grandchild's clothes." Frances lived on, inside of the inside of her apartment, in a city that could have been any city or any place anywhere or everywhere all the time, any time. In the parameters of her existence, she continued, as she always had, to be absorbed by a life that was for her in form and essence significant and purposeful.

Honey

That winter the first snowfall came early. It was just a dusting, but the sky was gray, the winds were forceful, the temperature had dropped into the teens, and the snow, which turned to rain and then back to snow, was steady. Suddenly, it felt like winter. Clara liked winter because it meant staying inside. There was no longer any pull to be outside; the cold weather made it inviting to be indoors. Winter brought internal rhythms, and like the animals who go into hibernation, digging holes in the ground and going under, Clara stayed at home in prayer and contemplation for long periods between November and March. Most evenings, she and Theo had a fire going. The front of the stove was glass so you could see the fire burning. It was the quietest of the four seasons and the snow absorbed the sounds into itself. Inside the cabin was peaceful, and Honey, the older cat, slept for hours on the cushion nearest the stove and worshipped the warmth.

Frances

When Frances was seventeen, she contemplated killing herself. It was during the war, and all around her were poverty and starvation. In her small town she was an outsider because she'd stopped going to church because she didn't believe in God or at least in the God that was feared by the priests and people who lived in her town. She lived with her mother. Her father had gone to France, originally for work, but ended up staying and not really working or making any earnings or sending any money back to the village in northern Italy, where Frances and her mother were starving. Eventually, Frances, worn out mainly by hunger, planned her suicide. She would go to the pharmacy, buy rat poison, take it, and lie down in the river. These were thoughts she had often, but they were particularly strong one day on her way home from school, and she decided to take the poison the next day. But when she got home, her mother greeted her with an unusual hopefulness, "Look what I found today," she said. She opened her hand to reveal a small morsel of food.

When Frances thought of what her mother must have done to get this food, thoughts of suicide left her mind completely. Her mother was a big woman who liked to eat. For Frances to watch her mother starve, knowing her mother had a big appetite ("she could eat three bowls of soup"), and to receive this little piece of food from her in the midst of their starvation, made a lasting impact on Frances. From then on, although she did not return to the church, her belief in her mother became a source of faith in goodness, and for the rest of her life she was always able to see the good in others even when it was hard. If she heard that someone was out of work or learned of someone's depression, hunger, illness, or demoralization, she prayed (as it turned out) to God to make things better. Later in her life, there wasn't a day when Frances didn't speak of this event.

Clara

The fire inside, orange; the snow outside, white. Orange and white. The sky gray, blanketed even at night due to the reflection of snow.

Sometimes there were intense winds. They came mostly from the mountains blowing in an easterly direction toward the river; but there were times when the winds blew in all directions at the same time. The little cabin where Clara and Theo lived was eighty years old and originally was used as a summer cottage and not a year-round house. After experiencing one of the coldest winters in a long time, with winds blowing at high speeds outside that could be felt blowing through the inside, Clara and Theo had insulation put in between the indoor and outdoor walls. This meant that no matter how high the speed of the winds outside, inside, the cabin was not windy.

As the end of the year approached, each day became shorter, darker, and colder. These increments for the most part were gradual, especially the timings of day and night, with the shifting of the rising and setting of the sun. Clara felt the absence of one less minute of light or the presence of one extra minute of darkness, so that while it was only a minute and the transition from long summer days to the short days of winter was gradual, the gradualness of it was not overlooked, and for every small or subtle transition, she was there as a witness.

Living in nature, Clara was aware not only of obvious changes like a tree with green leaves that turns to gold, or a tree full of leaves that turns into one with hardly any leaves, two leaves, and then none, but also watching within this, while it was happening, the first marks of red appearing on a green leaf, then a little more and more until at a certain point the leaf is more red than green, gradually transitioning itself into a completely different color. Clara watched fall disappear, and in doing so by the time it reached the quiet season of winter—the time to be inside, to put the storm windows up and be thankful for the insulation, to gaze at the glow of the embers in the stove and each day have the ritual of emptying out the tray of ash from under where the wood burns—by the time snow was on the ground and the car was hard to get to, Clara was in a fast lane to go nowhere, which was where she most wanted to go, against the out-going tide, inside.

Adam

Meanwhile Adam, who spent most of his time inside no matter what the season was, was practicing a moving meditation of shifting his weight from the right foot to the left foot while standing. The problem was that while he was doing this he was thinking of Ivy Lily who had had to go back to China where she was from, and leave him to live alone in Coney Island, staring out at the ocean and its waves and seeing only her. When he opened his kitchen cupboard and saw the bags of white rice and spices that she had cooked with, he lost his appetite as he found it difficult to eat without her. When he sat down to meditate, images of her laughing, sleeping, or cleaning came up in his mind so that he gave up on his meditations. In his loneliness and without his practices, he became strange. His neighbors worried about him and prayed for Ivy Lily's return.

Clara

When the winds blew in all directions Clara wondered if it had anything to do with her mind, how her thoughts jumped from one to another, each so different from the previous one. She wondered what a pure thought was. Watching her thoughts come and go was like watching clouds pass through the sky. She was familiar with both the sky and the landscape. She had taken walks in the mountains of northern India, during the winter when for a fleeting moment the cloud cover would open to reveal the Himalayas.

She experienced the transparency of the waveless lake and in it the reflection of birch trees. She stood before the paintings in the museums that spoke to her, transfixed by their beauty, leaving her with nothing to do and nowhere to go. She had entered through a door into a realm that provided stability so that her wanderings came momentarily to an end. She accepted that poetry was a way of describing a pure thought and that a pure thought could encompass one or many points. She realized that colors helped her to see, and dedicated moments of her life to admiring orange and green and thought of the oranges and apples that she had seen or tasted. She allowed for vividness and radiance to take control of her thoughts and her experience of this left her feeling renewed. Once again and always she understood Mother Nature as the creator and provider of squash, turmeric, cucumber, kale, water, and wheat.

Emmet

Emmet had a special vase that was given to him by a friend named Arthur who owned a high-end antique shop in Manhattan. When Emmet stopped by the shop one day to visit Arthur, though he could not see he went directly through the store to a table where the vase was the centerpiece and picked it up. For Emmet saw things by holding them, and in his grasp of extraordinary beauty, Arthur wanted to give him the vase despite the fact that at that time it was the most valuable object in the shop.

The vase was tall, narrow, ceramic, and white, with one black hand-drawn line running from top to bottom. It had a strange, uneven, or off-kilter look and feel to it, which things of the past that are handmade or weathered often have. The white of the vase was discolored and in some places pale yellow and other places pale gray. These variations were what made the vase one-of-a-kind. If one had wanted to make a duplicate, it would not have been possible.

In summer, Emmet used the vase for flowers. Often he collected flowers that attracted bees. He felt the company of the world through flowers and bees, who did not question his handicap or blindness or any other passing quality or circumstance of his. For him, the flowers (*les fleurs*, for he spoke and often thought in French) only asked of him that he appreciate them, and that he did. In winter, he gathered dried grasses and fallen tree branches and made arrangements out of them. Even when the vase was empty, in between one bouquet and another, it had a purpose in that it held the potential to hold what might come but had not come yet, as well as holding the memories of the past accumulations of hand-picked gatherings of flowers, plants, and grasses.

On occasion, the vase needed washing. Because it was large, his sink tiny, the vase precious, and Emmet blind, this task took his full attention.

He wouldn't think of daydreaming while washing the vase. In fact, it was after his fall, when he had to handle the vase so carefully, that he felt he saw it better. After years, he still appreciated it and kept it clean and felt that, even if it was an inanimate object, it had a substratum: a material, elemental, claylike, bone-like quality that was indescribable, unpredictable, distinct, and of a common substance.

Gloria

Many visiting teachers came through the school where Clara taught in New York City. It had become a meeting place for those who in the midst of a bustling metropolis crowded with people wanted time and space to be quiet and experience the mood of reflection. Clara was honored to teach there and made many friends through her work at the school. There was a certain amount of unpredictability as to who might be attracted to the school, and it seemed that people on cosmic levels would unexpectedly drop in. That's how it was when Gloria arrived.

Gloria was approaching a hundred and twenty years old and had long white hair she wore in a braid down her back. Her clothes were all orange— symbolic of the fire she had once burned all of her belongings in; symbolic of the life of renunciation. At the age of seven, she had had a vision of a statue of Quan Yin. She decided that the compassion she saw in the goddess was what she wanted for herself and then and there decided to become a sannyasin, a renunciate, and forgo marriage, children, and family life.

For many years, she lived in upstate New York, in the countryside in an ashram with other sannyasins. Gloria's main practice was meditation, which was what she taught. She said it was like climbing up the highest mountain, looking down, and seeing it all. From that viewpoint every-thing made sense. You could see life unfolding, as it had to, one event leading to the next, a divine order, people learning from their mistakes, making right and left turns, experiencing the pairs of opposites—sorrow and joy, love and hate, success and failure, health and illness—as they had to be experienced, as they were the two ends of the same road, as she saw it, from the cosmic level.

The vitality and richness of the emotions and complexities that people went through matured and this was how it was. Each event was part of a larger sequence and from the viewpoint of her meditations this was clear. She saw the picture and the pieces, the flower and its petals, at the same time. She understood the whys and the wherefores of how things came to be and where they were going, and for these reasons never judged anyone by a single act because there was no such thing as a single act. With the vision of all that came before, there would, through that understanding, always be a lot of compassion. Her mind was at rest. She had focused on a single object long enough, since the moment she had decided to become like Quan Yin. She had never thought to herself that she couldn't do it. She had never canceled herself out.

Gloria heard voices in her meditations and dreams. These voices were her teachers and at times in her life when her teachers were not physically nearby, she always heard these voices and never felt alone. Over time, the teachings that she heard came from all directions from plants, animals, and people with or without languages that she knew or did not know, so that she was always in communication with subtle vibrations, made up of sounds, voices, and cries. She knew if a dog had died or was nearing death, in a house that she passed by. She knew what day people would arrive to visit her, before they even planned on coming. She heard trees crying while they were chopped down, and when people spoke to her in their own languages, she understood, never needing a translator. She was not impatient for her enlightenment. She knew she had been waiting for a long time and that it would come. She understood that it was more than a cup of coffee she was waiting for. She was childlike and mature and could see backward, forward, and far into time. She was not afraid of running out of time, nor was she burdened by time. The world was transparent.

Clara

Clara was sure she had been a dog in a past life, which explained her fear of thunder. Lucy said she was certain she was dark-skinned in a past life and it was for this reason that the first boy she kissed was African. Das said he was certain he had known Clara before in a previous life, and that made her happy. Clara thought it was possible that lifetimes ago Meryl had actually been her daughter, Theo a brother, Madeleine a sister, Das a close confidant: so that the idea that they were all in each other's lives before, perhaps even more than once, in different capacities, made sense to Clara. If she could see far enough into the past or future, these changes in the outer forms of her relationships would become clear. Until then, it was a feeling she had that most people she knew she'd known before, reappearing in infinite ways, and that even when she met someone "new," she recognized them as someone from her past, or someone she knew all along she'd meet in her future. She recognized the seeds and cycles of flowers, some cut, others left to grow wild, some in vases, others in the woods or on the roadside, some picked, pulled, admired, or perished quickly by a sudden cool frost or a heavy rain, like a cloud or bird passing by and parting.

Ling

Ling, Clara's neighbor, belonged to a Buddhist sect known as the Pure Land. The Pure Land referred to a mental landscape, free of the capacity to harm. Out of this landscape one could read the mental landscapes of others. There were no obstructions or biases that cause agitations or misunderstandings. Communication was subtle and yet, as subtle can be, transformative. At times, Clara felt like she was momentarily there in the Pure Land and then just when she felt it, it was gone, for it took a lot of meditation to stay there. It was said that when someone was in the presence of a bodhisattva who lived in the Pure Land, they were transparent to the bodhisattva. This enabled the one not in the Pure Land to glimpse what the one in the Pure Land saw.

Gloria

One of the things about Gloria was that not everyone could see her. She could decide to whom she would or would not appear before. Through her meditations, she could remove all the density or materiality of her body so that all that was left was transparency and light, so that if you were sitting somewhere and out of nowhere something started to shimmer or glow, it might have been Gloria. She was drawn to dark places as it was there she felt most needed, traveling through the ether, appearing materially when necessary: bringing food to children hiding in basements of cities in countries in upheaval; making her way through areas of danger without any danger to her since she was not visible until she arrived where the children were, with food and sometimes blankets, soap or light bulbs, and became visible again. Such was the power behind her meditations.

Gazelle

Gazelle, perhaps because she had grown up in the midst of war and therefore uncertainty, had an uncanny way of reading signs, so that, wherever she was, some good would come out of the situation. One holiday season she decided not to go home to the Middle East to be with her family.

Purchasing an airplane ticket for the days she wanted to fly seemed unusually difficult and expensive, so she felt in some way that she was not meant to go. It was then decided, since she wasn't going home and was staying in New York instead, that she would go to the mansion that had once belonged to Marigold's grandmother. Since her grandmother's passing, Marigold's mother was living there and Marigold spent a lot of time visiting and often gave parties, especially around the holidays, when she invited people who for one reason or another weren't going back home. Everyone loved these parties. It was fun to be in a mansion that was actually quite cozy, inviting, and even a bit messy and neglected in ways that made everyone feel at home. The particular year that Gazelle decided not to go home and instead go the party at the mansion, Marigold's father died, and Marigold cried all night on the bed with Gazelle there, also equally heartbroken, for that is how Gazelle is. Everyone thought it was such a blessing that that particular year Gazelle had stayed back and was there to comfort Marigold through the darkest hours of the night, in which her father, who loved her probably more than anyone else, passed.

✿ ✿ ✿

One time when Clara was teaching at a retreat center in Vermont, Gazelle, having had a dream where Clara was drowning, woke up and decided at the last minute to go to the teachings. After the weekend of teachings, Clara and Gazelle headed back to New York City but they never made it because the rains were so heavy. Clara couldn't see to drive so they ended up staying in a hotel that had a restaurant in its lobby where they sat drinking wine and tea and celebrating their friendship. Clara was not a good driver and was easily upset by heavy rains. So, on that night with Gazelle, who suggested and probably even paid for the hotel, Clara was filled with relief and affection, the relief and affection that Gazelle's life and timing seemed to bring to so many.

Whereas people observe the land and watch as seeds sprout and turn into a plant that flowers; whose seeds are eaten by birds who fly to distant lands carrying the potential for new flower seeds—all in a rhythm of seasons and time, with its mini-rhythms and rhythms within rhythms, quick and slow, affected by winds and weather, understanding transformations, interdependence, growth, and change, all from observing the fruition of a seed—Gazelle watched war and death lead to more deaths, to retaliation, revenge, side-taking, and hatred. Through all that she saw, she always asked herself what it would take to stop this. Her power to discern cause and effect, even if there were great gaps between the two (as there sometimes are), became strong. In the watching of worlds mature, of seeds or war or both, it is possible to predict way before the end what the end will be. Gazelle looked for signs and recognized them when they appeared, as messages foretelling what was to come.

She knew beforehand when someone would die, and because of that, inevitably, she would be with those who loved her at the time of their departure. On one occasion, at the last minute, without really knowing why, she canceled a trip to Argentina. Two days later she was holding Adrienne's young hand as he was dying, in a hospital bed, having been diagnosed with an extremely aggressive form of stomach cancer literally three weeks before. When she herself passed (decades later for she lived to be over a hundred), no kind word had been left unsaid, no debt unpaid. Everything was in order—exemplifying the life of someone whose life had had meaning and whose ups and downs were always symbolic of a greater picture. Her circle was large and always increasing, full of those who wanted her company. It wasn't only because she had lived through war that she was good company, but that her having lived through war had somehow enlightened her understanding of the preciousness of friendship. If she was in a cab on her way to the airport she would call a friend to say, "I'm in a cab on my way to the airport," and the friend would feel that it was special to be thought of by Gazelle in her travels. She never overlooked how powerful small exchanges of this sort between friends are. She had no hostility, she was not demanding, she did not criticize or judge . . . she harmonized and inspired, and everyone loved her.

Frances

When Frances was seventeen she left her home in Italy to be a housekeeper for a wealthy family in England. Mostly she sewed and embroidered clothes, curtains, tablecloths, linens, etc., for the lady of the house, Mrs. Barr. Mrs. Barr, who hadn't had children and was lonely, took a liking to Frances and taught her English by virtue of conversation, mainly in the evenings. One strong memory Frances had was Mrs. Barr telling her about her sister, who'd died from a rare disease around the time of her menopause. Her sister had been a poet and one of her poems that Mrs. Barr recited frequently was about a donkey that no one appreciated. Everyone thought the donkey was stupid and just used it as a working animal, frightening and forcing the donkey to carry things. The poem told the story of a man, humiliated and frustrated by his poverty and the poverty around him, who befriended this gentle donkey, who was equally humiliated and hungry.

The creations of Frances were extraordinary: she embroidered monograms on all the sheets and towels; she covered all the pillows with cases that she'd hand-stitched pictures on depicting the English landscape; she made and designed all the clothes, hats, and purses for Mrs. Barr; and came up with elaborate patterns using flower and bird motifs. For that she was well paid, especially considering her background and the hardships of most people in Europe at that time. Though Mrs. Barr loved her and her work, for Frances at her age it was not enough.

She became anxious, had difficulty sleeping, and suffered from fevers and chills. Living there she became, like Mrs. Barr, lonely. Mrs. Barr took her to a variety of doctors, clinics, and specialists who all said there was nothing wrong with her, but she knew she would have to leave England and go back home.

Mrs. Barr gave Frances enough money to travel back to Italy, but somehow she lost some of it or it was stolen and virtually penniless she ended up in France where at least she spoke the language. She slept in the shelter connected to the railway station and every day she went to the job agency in search of work. She couldn't get a job because she didn't have the right papers, and she couldn't get the papers because she didn't have a job, and so she felt she was caught in a vicious cycle. Each day that she went to the job agency and was turned away without a job, she became more desperate, until one day all she had left was two subway tokens and her coat, which she figured she could sell if she had to.

On that day, the man at the job agency told her, "I see you here every day." The man had a job for her: a mother was looking for someone to look after her kids because she and her husband were dancers and traveled a lot. They weren't looking for someone with experience necessarily but rather someone "nice." The man said, "You look like a nice person." He telephoned the mother and described Frances, "She is kind, compassionate, honest, and hard-working." This description, based on seeing her for a few minutes over a few days, couldn't have been more accurate. Frances got the job and on account of it traveled to America with the couple, their kids, and the whole dance company. When the couple went back to France, she stayed and got married. So much of her life had happened because of this man who'd seen something dignified in her that made him want to help her. She thought about him often and told this story, of how she got the job with the dancers and came to America all on account of this man. And every time she told it she cried and said it was a miracle.

Sun

Sun's name was not originally Sun. Her friends started calling her that because of her interest in solar gods and the solar system and because she worshipped the sun's graceful movement across the sky. She even came up with a set of movements to formally honor and greet the sun. She organized her prayers around the time of sunrise and sunset, and felt at those times that she was traveling through a transition of light. For Sun, darkness was the sun's quiet period, offering the moon and stars the foreground as it disappeared for a while into the background until it reemerged. Out of these cycles came day and night, life and death, and light and dark, giving her the opportunity to experience her days as rhythmic and musical. There was a time, toward the end of her life, when she went into the forest for seven months, making a bed out of oak leaves and pine needles, twigs and grasses. She had a small clock she relied on for knowing the time and she used it to structure her days. But soon after the first month passed, the clock broke.

While this upset her at first, eventually it gave her a sense of freedom and encouraged her to follow time by following the sun directly. In this way she learned that when the sunlight was in between the two nearby hills it would be the middle of the day, and this was the best time for her to have her main meal. This time, without time, without a clock, was a happy one, for it was during this time as well as at other times that she used her time well.

After Eli passed away, Clara could not telephone him with questions about the solar systems, so it was Sun that she went to with her questions. What Sun and Eli studied about the galaxies varied: Sun was a poet and primarily interested in spirituality, and Eli was a physicist and placed an emphasis on science. Both were passionate about their interests and they both stayed awake all night if there was an eclipse, meteor showers, or shooting stars.

Sun's reverie was over the way the disc of the moon appeared illuminated and how this appearance of illumination caused by the sun's light was always changing, so that the shape of the light part of the moon caused the moon to appear different, waxing and waning as it was. She noticed that where the moon was in its cycle affected her moods; she often felt a little overwhelmed when the moon was full. She understood the moon's effect on the ocean's tides as motion, gravity, and balance in the Earth–moon system, pulling things together and apart, including herself, as an art form.

Eli

Eli understood the science behind the moon's illumination, the highs and lows of the tides and the cycles of the sun, moon, Earth, and stars. He knew how and why the stars placed themselves as they did. All through his eighties, when he was frail and no longer left the house, he did from time to time spend the night outside in the back yard in order to watch the sky, even if it was November or January when he could be cold. He knew how to calculate how far away from Earth the stars were by their brightness and could organize their orbit in his mind, such that he did not (like most scientists) need a telescope.

He knew the comets, clouds, orbits, asteroids and galaxies, gases and dust, numbers, formulas, planets, sounds, colors, and pulsations of rivers and rocks. He understood magnetics and the pull of gravity and that he was made up of the same elements as nature. The movements of the sun, moon, and stars corresponded with his own movements, so that when the sky seemed particularly auspicious it was in relation to internal auspices, within a world within himself, so that Eli saw that his enteric nervous system (the nervous system around his navel), primitive as it was, was a link to a much vaster system, and that behind those systems lay infinite possibilities. These thoughts of Eli's were shared with Sun, and this was why the movements that Sun had pieced together to make herself attractive to the solar gods included turnings of the waist, which brought an awareness of the subtle energy that traveled through the channels linked to the digestive system yet were not limited to digestion as its only function.

Through practice, Sun had the experience of feeling her memories and emotions stored in these places and that it was important not to obstruct those channels with too much food, or the wrong food. She remained throughout her life narrow-waisted, and this is symbolic of an unburdened system and thereby a life that was free of many of the problems that weigh most people down. She was actually often not hungry or even thirsty for long periods of time because she said she was "nourished by the celestial deities." What this meant was that often she was in a special state of mind such that though she was always grateful for any tiny amount of food, though she was a great cook who had created a wide variety of recipes as simple as they were delicious, and though she always offered the food first to the Divine, eating or drinking and all the work it involved was an activity she often skipped. Of course, some people thought she should eat more and were concerned, but since she was never short on energy and always looked her best, it seemed that she knew what she was doing.

Tiffany

At the age of twenty-two, Tiffany wanted to study with Clara, but her study could not take place because she was sick all the time. No one knew exactly what was wrong with her. She had seen many doctors and had been given different diagnoses and treatments, but by the time she was twenty-five she couldn't even walk down the street. Most of the time she was living with her parents, which was not a great situation as her father drank and her mother had chronic depression. Nonetheless, Tiffany, who couldn't work or earn any livelihood for herself, was loved by her parents, and she was a good influence in the house, especially on her younger brother. Though it was difficult for her to live there, there was purpose in it, too.

Tiffany prayed often and (according to her) her prayers were being answered all the time. She believed her sickness and all that it entailed was the Divine's way of teaching her to cultivate the right virtues for her enlightenment: so that when she could no longer take part in the activities that she had loved and spent most of her life doing—such as singing, dancing, and hanging out with friends—she saw this as an opportunity to go deep into meditation such that she withdrew herself from the world, like a tortoise retracting its head into its shell.

Tiffany lived quietly in her room, the same room she had lived in as a healthy and active teenager, resting her mind on the Divine. She offered the small things: the way she kept her room clean or made the occasional phone call or looked out of the window to see what the weather was. She tried to do everything she could thoughtfully, no matter how small, and attributed this desire to Clara, whom she said had taught her this and thereby opened many doors. Tiffany had the ability to accept her sickness with equanimity, in moments when she felt better and in moments when she felt worse, so that though she'd had to give up so much she was not unhappy.

One night she dreamt that she was standing by the side of a river. In her dream she knew the river to be symbolic of travel. When she walked in the water and the waves carried her on her journey, she had the feeling she was leaving her illness behind. When she awoke, she knew that she would have to leave her surroundings in order to get well. It was an intuition that came like a flash of light and in her heart she knew that the dream was a sign for her to follow.

Three weeks later, with the help of her younger brother, she traveled to Mont Blanc, the highest mountain in the Alps, to be with a holy woman, one with special powers, who was seen by her followers as a servant of the Goddess and considered a great healer. She treated Tiffany over a period of three months and during that time Tiffany had many visions of angels all around her. Much of the time, Tiffany prayed for the wellbeing of others—her parents, of course, but also the sick people around her, who like herself had left their homes to place themselves in the care of this special healer, who with her higher abilities for hearing, touching, seeing, tasting, and smelling, would use her senses and in collaboration with the divine force she served bring Tiffany and the others back to health.

While Tiffany was in Europe she was taught to meditate and in these meditations to try to distinguish between a thought she had around her illness, and the actual illness, as well as who she was without the illness. This was important because she'd grown so used to thinking of herself as a sick person that at times she'd lost a greater sense of who she was. She was also encouraged in these meditations to persevere, especially when she wasn't feeling well, which was often, when it was hard for her even to swallow.

Clara

Clara first traveled to India when she was twenty-one. She made friends with Anita, who was older and more mature. Anita was from Lübeck, Germany, where Thomas Mann was born and where Anita lived and worked as a nurse. Anita had made several trips to India before and had traveled all over Southeast Asia. Clara and Anita met in a restaurant that was crowded and they ended up sharing a table. They spoke of India and realized that their reasons for being there were similar. They enjoyed each other's company and both agreed that at that time, the late 1980s, it was difficult as a woman to be traveling alone. That year and at that time of year, it was especially hot, so hot that even the local people stayed indoors at mid-day. Anita and Clara were happy spending the hot part of the day sitting in the restaurant drinking club sodas with lime. When they were leaving, Anita asked Clara if she wanted to go with her to the temple on the outskirts of town. There was a priest she wanted to see. Clara was lonely as she had been traveling for months by herself, and she was happy to leave the restaurant with Anita.

Together, Anita and Clara went to the temple where the priest greeted them pleasantly. He knew Anita from before. He taught them both a simple exercise that involved breathing in through one nostril and out through the other. Clara liked the way it made her feel . . . balanced. The priest said that this exercise could be practiced every day for five to ten minutes and would bring great results. After the lesson, he spoke about himself. He had been married and had a grown daughter. He became a priest after the unexpected death of his wife. How she died he did not say but his daughter was living in New Jersey and it was obvious that he missed her a lot. He invited them to stay for the lunch he would be making. He explained that he had his own avocado tree and that he knew different ways to prepare avocados: raw, boiled, fried, prepared as a sweet or a savory, etc. He was a kind man, curious about Anita and Clara, and when they were leaving he asked Clara for her address and told them both to keep in touch. They could tell he was sincere.

As time passed, Anita went back to Germany and Clara back to traveling by herself in northern India. Wherever she went, every morning for five to ten minutes and often longer she practiced what she'd learned from the priest. One morning, she left her room and went up on the rooftop of the hotel where she was staying. It was the time of day the priest had recommended: dawn. The city was quiet, the traffic had not yet begun, and it seemed as if only the crows and Clara were up. Sitting on the rooftop, Clara inhaled through the left nostril and exhaled through the right; inhaled through the right and exhaled through the left. She did this back and forth for several minutes when she heard a door open and footsteps; she knew that she was no longer alone. She opened her eyes just enough to see a man and child nearby. She closed her eyes and continued with her breathing. The child asked his father what it was that the lady was doing.

Though he was whispering, Clara heard the father say, "She's praying." The father told the child that they should go back downstairs so as not to disturb her. She heard their footsteps get quieter as they walked further away from her and eventually back downstairs. There she was, left on the rooftop, praying. She had not known she was praying until then, but after the man and child went downstairs everything about what she was doing changed. She sat like that for a while, not really knowing for how long. But when she came out of it, the day was on its way, you could hear the traffic, and it was already starting to get hot. She thought of the priest and felt, without herself ever having lost a spouse, the loss of his wife as if it were her own. It was like she knew what it felt like without it actually having happened to her.

* * *

Occasionally, there were days that Clara and Theo especially enjoyed, in that on these days neither of them had anywhere to go or anything necessary to do. These days usually coincided with a steady light rain, snow falling, or the new moon. On these days, Theo would tell Clara what he was reading and the two of them would drink tea—Theo green, and Clara black with almond milk and sugar. Clara was always interested in what Theo was reading and her desire to hear how he felt about what he was reading prompted within Theo powerful insights while he told her the stories, and these stories reminded him and her of other stories. In this way, they could pass the day recollecting events that they had both read about and experienced.

On one such day, Theo was telling Clara about a meeting that took place between a young blind girl and an older black man on a park bench. The girl was blind because her mother had in a fit of anger thrown a knife across the room and into her face. The black man was not accustomed to speaking or sitting with anyone white, as segregation was prevalent at the time and place of the story. But since the girl was blind, she was innocent of his color. The girl sat on this bench most afternoons and used her time there as a way of getting away from her mother and the general dysfunction and negativity of her home. They were outcasts, him being black and she being blind, and both were alone. Somehow, there were no mental limitations in the way of their understanding one another. From the moment they spoke to each other there was a trust, more in her because she couldn't see him, but he could identify with her immediately. They felt a platonic love for each other and began meeting secretly in the park. While Theo told Clara this story, she was thinking what a good man Theo was, and it was clear to her that he lived under the influence of goodness and that his actions came out of the same quality of feeling that existed between the blind girl and the black man.

Isaac

Isaac, whom no one knew really well and who'd lived in the same town his whole life, said he could levitate. The people who knew him did not believe him, so one day he told them he would show them over the weekend. The word spread, so that what was originally planned as a small viewing turned into a larger one. Clara, who lived on the same street as Isaac, planned to go.

Isaac lived in a small brick house with his wife, Martha, and their eight cats. Most of their furniture had been transformed by the cats, who slept inside of the fortresses they made out of the inner linings of the two couches that faced each other in the living room. Isaac and Martha had their own resourceful and primitive ways of supplying themselves with heat, hot water, and electricity. They gardened all summer and tapped maple trees in the winter for syrup. They were easy-going people, and when the cats started tearing apart the couches they didn't make any attempts to stop them.

Their house was placed in the middle of their garden, which had numerous pathways and a small pond with lilies and lotuses growing out of the water. Everything was overgrown and meandering, untidy and muddy, and beautiful in a wild way. Isaac and Martha didn't have a lot of land, but the bushes and shrubs were so close together, and grew so high, that they ended up having a lot of privacy. The levitation was to take place behind their house, next to the pond in the late afternoon just before dusk. It was a fine summer day. Everyone gathered and sat down, awaiting the expected event.

Once they were quiet, Isaac stood in front of them and closed his eyes. He stood like that for a few minutes with his eyes closed and his body still and it created a mood of suspense—until finally he began singing. He sang to them a simple song about the perfection of the day, perfect because they were together and assembled in one place: his back yard. Collectively, they could uplift each other and set their problems aside. He kept repeating, "Today is a perfect day." Everyone was fascinated, and as Isaac sang his neighbors quietly settled down and became transfixed by the singing and by Isaac. The light started changing as the sun was going down and everyone's spirits were raised.

Isaac was good looking and had a thick neck or no real jaw line and his bottom lip turned in. His eyes were slanted and his glasses extra thick. While he sang, his gaze was turned slightly upward, just above everyone's heads. His clothes were torn and dirty because he'd been outside working. All of these slight peculiarities endeared those who had come to see him levitate.

Many of the people there that night described Isaac as radiant. People said that even in the dark they could see him glowing. Some said they saw an aura of light around his head. They said his song was unlike any other and no one could have imagined how talented he was. They said he could have been an opera singer; he sounded otherworldly, it was haunting, and he took their breath away. During the song, Clara all of a sudden felt the presence of Wise One pervading the space around her, and when the singing stopped and it was dark and silent, Wise One was there, distinct but intangible, just to the left of her shoulder. Of course, she often thought of and pictured Wise One in her mind, but this experience was different; it was not connected to her normal projections or imagery. It was awesome and lasted for more than a few minutes. Then Wise One disappeared through the sky and into the horizon. It seemed that everyone had experienced something—faith perhaps, goodness, song, community—such that the need for proof that the neighbors had come with was released and love was in the atmosphere. The evening dissolved and everyone went home, elevated, light as cotton, and so weightless that they walked on water across the pond and then through the air as well.

Theo

Theo came home after a long day of hard work complaining that the ulcer in his patient's foot had become infected because the dressing wasn't changed often enough. Theo's world at the hospital was full of people with bodies that had mostly been uncared for: people who'd smoked all their lives, drank excessively, ate poorly, and had a lot of emotional problems that led to many stress factors and lifestyles that were destructive. The bodies that he looked at and touched were bruised, inflamed, bloated, and unhealthy. Theo, who tried to make his patients more comfortable and tried up to a point to educate them, did not judge them. Clara admired this quality of his, which came naturally to him, as it was clear to him that one's Self was not the body, that the Self lived independent of the body, and that one needed to look beyond the body to see the Self inside. It was because almost everyone misunderstood this that people for the most part walked around feeling confined, even alien.

Theo understood the relationship between the elements and the senses, and was always bringing what he thought would help his patients in the way of food or music that tasted or sounded particularly wonderful, or would simply make time to hold their hand or massage them so they could be touched. All of this affected his patients, and especially in Theo's presence it put them in a mood where their minds could conceive of the possibility that there was a soul, spirit, or purpose not limited to their bodies, which were falling apart.

Not only did Theo sit in communion with the eternal soul of a patient, he also understood the mechanics of a body: how organs functioned, fluids filtered, and the heart pumped. He knew digestion to be the fire element; bones, the earth element; blood, the water element; and breath, the wind element. He concentrated well on these elements and meditated on what their commonality was. If Theo was your nurse, you were in good hands.

Though Theo was thin and sometimes felt fragile and didn't have the physical strength that some of the men around him had (nor the education, as he'd gone through an abbreviated form of nursing school that took only two years, where he had a minimum of academic requirements compared with other nursing programs), none of that seemed to matter when it came to his ability to take care of others. If he needed to lift someone much heavier than he, if it would help a patient to sit in a chair and get out of the bed, he could effortlessly pick the patient up and set him or her back down in a comfortable position. If he had a patient who couldn't speak, didn't know English, was traumatized, or had a tube going down their throat, he could discern what they wanted, and what they would say, if they could. If he had a patient who was yelling at him, cursing, even violent, he could win favor with them mainly because he wasn't concerned with winning favor with them; he was only concerned with their well-being.

Sometimes, without anyone knowing how, he could treat several patients at the same time. One patient would say, "Yes, he was just here bandaging my foot"; another would say, "Yes, he was just here massaging my hand"; and another would say, "He was just here giving me a shave." What was even more odd was that his mother Frances, who lived several hours away from the hospital where Theo worked, would say, "He was just here fixing my bathtub," or "He just brought me the *New York Times.*" It seemed that if anyone in a crisis situation thought of Theo, he would appear and help them.

When Theo came home from work from his hard day of ulcers, amputations, and infections, he enjoyed eating walnuts or a thinly sliced piece of toast or a sliver of chocolate cake with a glass of wine. He hung out with the cats, Honey and Hazel, and listened to music—jazz or classical. Sometimes if it was jazz, he would dance to it or pretend he was playing the trumpet or drums or whatever instrument was especially featured, and this would make Clara laugh. Sometimes he would take a walk and look at the leaves, trees, and grasses, and say *hello* to the neighboring dog.

Theo took such pleasure in these relatively small endeavors because his senses were so refined and he never prided himself for his work, or for anything really. He never thought of himself as the doer. He was an instrument, a flute or violin or trumpet, in the hands of a spirit that was moving through an orchestra. He was a small composition in a symphony, one he knew himself to be a part of and one he knew was part of himself. None of this could be explained or described in words. It was evoked and hinted at in his movements, when he danced the tango with his eyes closed.

Wise One

When Wise One was at the end of his life, he couldn't remember much of the many scriptures he'd memorized and keenly studied. He couldn't remember the basic vocabulary or philosophy of what he'd taught to so many over most of his life. He couldn't remember the names or even the faces of his students—even the close ones, such as those who returned to India year after year and sat at his feet and learned from him—and later from his family. He forgot to eat. He forgot that he was a great and revered man who'd traveled the world and amassed a large sum of money, which he gave generously to build temples and hospitals throughout southern India.

However, he did remember his wife of sixty years, whose death came ten years before his, and he usually remembered to put a flower by the picture of his teacher that he kept at his bedside. He remembered God . . . or it wasn't really that he remembered God, for that would imply some kind of effort, the effort to remember. It was more that, since he'd forgotten most everything else, his mind was free, his life uncluttered, and his time infinite. Wise One was peaceful about all the things he forgot. He experienced none of the humiliations that most people feel around aging, loss, and death, and this became his final teaching—his ease with it all.

Clara got to be with him in this state several times. His diabetes had become so bad that his vision was blurry and he was always thirsty. The diabetes led to other serious problems, so that he had a lot of nerve pain and difficulty digesting his food and kept dropping weight. He fell a lot and was often bleeding. While at times it was hard for Clara or many of the many people around him to see him this way, it was not hard for him to be seen this way. He was happy. He was somewhere else, here and there simultaneously. He knew the body and soul were different in nature and quality and distinguished between that which changes and that which is changeless, and it was within the changeless that he resided. There was physical pain to be experienced, but the one experiencing the pain knew himself to be other than the pain, as pain belonged to the world of change, of comings and goings, and Wise One identified with the eternal.

Wise One had grown up in a small village where the people worshipped many gods and demigods who lived in realms, some of which were demonic and dark and others benevolent and bright. It was believed that at any time, but especially around the time of death, an emanation from one of these realms would find a way to influence the one who was dying, so that they would desire entry into one of those realms, whether demonic or benevolent. Of course, it would be better to go to a benevolent realm, but these were still the realms of gods and demigods and so they were seen as less than the Supreme that existed beyond these realms.

It was also believed that if the one dying desired to go to such a realm, this final desire or attachment would impede their emancipation because their death would not have been desireless. Because of this, usually the family members around the dying recited prayers that the one who was passing wouldn't get detoured into one of these realms and that there wouldn't be any last desires, attractions, or influences, so that he or she would be free to merge in the Absolute, Ultimate Supreme Being. But in Wise One's case, it was different. He was free of such influences and desires, was unclouded, clearheaded, and pure, and the priest of Wise One's village said that such prayers were not necessary and that this was extremely rare.

* * *

When Wise One left his body, the family began what would be days, weeks, months, and years of rituals, festivities, and celebrations all in relation to the time of his parting. Certain prayers would take place one day after, three days after, eleven days after, etc.; and then other rituals, the first new moon after, Tuesday after, full moon after, etc. Timings were considered very important and had to be exact. If one were to offer fruit to the deceased in the morning, it had to be before a certain time; and if the fruit on the altar had been inappropriately or mistakenly offered later, then later, by simply looking at the fruit, the family's priest, who knew that the prayers to protect Wise One from the influence of various emanations weren't necessary, also knew that the fruit (which looked like any other fruit) had not been offered at the right time.

Wise One, from a very early age, had lived a dedicated life. His desire was to take care of his family, study, worship, and teach, and that was how he spent his time, while remaining a humble man. He taught a practice that he'd learned from his teacher that cured people of their afflictions and blessed them with every success possible, so that when his students fulfilled their potential—leading joyous, rewarding, purposeful lives, and not wasting their time—they all knew it was Wise One who'd made this happen. There were hundreds if not thousands of students who felt immense gratitude for his presence in their life. Much of what he did, with a few words (for English was not his first language), a side-glance, or a firm push or pull (for he did teach through touch), had this lasting positive effect that was overwhelming. One wondered how it was that Wise One was able to have set so much in motion.

Despite his diabetes, Wise One liked his coffee sweet and rice salty. He enjoyed going to the market to buy vegetables or pretending to drink tea with his three-year-old granddaughter. If you came to his house carrying some sort of shopping bag, he wanted to know what was in it and would start taking the things out, examining them. When he stayed in a student's home while he was traveling as a guest teacher, he would open the closets and drawers, not to snoop but to better know where he was. He would pick things up to further his understanding and then put them back such that the object seemed to the student more valuable than before, partly because Wise One had touched it but also because when he was holding the object—a picture, a vase, a book, or piece of fruit—the object appeared different and took on new meaning. This was the beauty of hanging out with Wise One . . . seeing through his eyes.

Wise One had the loveliest smile. He had swollen ankles, probably because of the diabetes, and also glaucoma, which made the color of his eyes shift back and forth from gray to blue to green. His eyeglasses were held together with duct tape and other times with string until finally one student took him to the eye doctor, who told him that the "specs" he had been wearing for decades were of "no use." He purchased a new gold pair, for he enjoyed gold as well as many other fine material objects, yet he was never attached to them. Nothing ever prevented him from his daily worship or teaching. He reached the highest states of absorption, and a sense of self as a separate entity no longer existed as real. Perhaps this was the reason that he could reach anyone, anywhere, anytime, as a benevolent force.

Book IV: The Rain Cloud

Clara

Clara's story would not exist had she not been born. While this is obvious, Clara never took it for granted. She knew that the scriptures said that birth in a body is necessary for one's enlightenment to take place. While commentaries on the scriptures have been written, full of explanations or descriptions of what would make for a good or bad birth, Clara herself of course did not know. She had seen her father, who was born in a place, time, and country where all of his relations were murdered, become a great scientist and a kind and gentle man.

It was said of the Buddha that even he had to leave his palace in order to see suffering and generate compassion. Many enlightened ones have had hard lives. Clara knew that Sun's upbringing was no piece of cake and had the idea that Sun had to assume a lot of responsibility in regard to things that most children don't have to take on. From an early age, Sun looked after herself. When she was sick, she cured herself. She remembers picking weeds on the roadside or in the yard, making medicines from them and feeling better—first out of necessity, and later, because she never trusted pharmaceuticals. She always recognized Mother Nature's bounty (weeds, grasses, and roots) as offerings to Earth's creatures for their wellbeing, and taught many around her to do the same. "How incredible it is," she would say, "that if you have a sore throat, you can gargle with turmeric and feel better." In this regard, she was like Lucy, who always had turmeric root on her altar. Lucy made a drink with homemade almond milk, turmeric, ginger, black pepper, cardamom, and maple syrup that was creamy and sweet and golden in color and cured just about anything.

Eli

In the last ten years of his life, Eli did not leave the house. He was afraid of falling, losing control of his bladder, and due to his swollen feet it had become difficult to wear shoes. He was comfortable at home and having lived nine decades there wasn't much that interested him outside of the house anymore. This does not mean there weren't people and places he would have gone had he been feeling better. He missed talking to the man from Mexico who sold fruit in a parking lot outside the shopping center. He missed his weekly meal at the diner—not so much for the food, for he always complained it was too salty, but he liked the waitress. Even when one waitress would leave and a new one was hired, he always got along well with waitresses.

He missed going to the temple on Sabbath, not because he liked the services particularly but because without going he didn't feel he was a good Jew. When he stopped going out, Eli and Sarah's social life decreased. It was around that time that Eli became interested in the music of Franz Schubert, in particular the song cycle known as *Winterreise*. The cycle uses a text taken from twenty-four poems written by the German poet Wilhelm Müller, who was born in 1794 and was the son of a shoemaker. The piece of music was written in 1827 for voice and piano.

During the time that Schubert wrote it, at the age of thirty, he was dying of syphilis and deeply depressed. This melancholia is reflected in the music, described as having a gloomy, dark, and tragic tone. But Eli found the music and its pathos comforting, and he understood German, so he knew what was being said in the songs. The poems were about a man disappointed in love. Having to leave his home, he sets out on a cold, snowy wintry night with no companion on a journey to where he does not know. Toward the end of his journey, he comes to a tree; underneath the boughs is a man playing the organ. The organ music is sad yet beautiful, but no one around him seems to hear the music or even notice the musician playing. Eli loved and listened to this piece of music over and over. There were different versions of it, as it has been interpreted differently over time; the vocal part was sometimes sung by a woman, but more often by a man.

All his life, memories of the war haunted Eli. Because of that, he had a way of looking at things so that he always imagined and predicted the worst. But finally at the end of his life, it was too tiring to be pessimistic all the time. Instead, he lay on the bed, closed his eyes, and listened to *Winterreise*. To see Eli lying in bed listening to music in the middle of the day and not slumped over his desk either working or sleeping was somewhat hard to take in, because he'd worked so hard his whole life. He had not been a lazy man.

Not that lying in bed and listening to music in the middle of the afternoon is the same as being lazy. Actually, the late pieces of Schubert are said to be quite demanding on the listener, and Schubert himself worked himself to exhaustion, never stopping, even when he was sick. When he completed one piece, he immediately set to work on another, becoming more and more ambitious and driven, each year of his short and (at the time) uncelebrated life. He died in Vienna, the same city he was born in; the same city of Eli's childhood until the time of war, when at age ten Eli fled to Czechoslovakia and from there traveled to America.

When Eli died, Clara was not at his bedside. She was far away on the other side of the country when she got a call from her brother Solon in the middle of the night, the time of night the phone never rings unless someone has died or come close to it. Solon said that Eli had died peacefully in his sleep, that the funeral would be in a couple of days, and that he and his family were already that morning on their way to the airport to fly to California, where Eli and Sarah had been living for the last ten years. Clara did not quite believe it, tried to shake it off like a bad dream, preoccupy herself with something else, go back to sleep, or try planning her class lessons . . . all to no avail.

What Clara wondered most about Eli's passing was whether or not he'd really died peacefully. There was the music, the simple meals of broccoli or vanilla ice cream, and the money in Vienna. These things would have been comforting to him. There was the natural wisdom that anyone with Eli's level of humility and kindness would have: knowledge greater than book learning, although he'd learned plenty through reading books and even in his nineties was reading Homer and Dante. There was the knowledge that Solon and Clara were happy and healthy and since Eli had chronic back-, stomach-, and chest-pain, death would bring relief from all of that. But underlying those things, Eli always had angst. It would probably have been worse had he not worked such long hours in his laboratory, been married to Sarah, or at the end of his life listened to Franz Schubert.

Clara gathered that the two main causes of his deep sorrow were his survivor's guilt, for he escaped Nazi Europe whereas many of his relations and friends did not, and the death of his mother at the age of forty-eight from having taken medicines that the doctor had prescribed for her during her menopause. These two tragedies were a big part of Eli's make-up and so it was rare that Eli with all of his great scientific insights and accomplishments really felt relaxed about himself or the world. So Clara wondered whether or not at the time of his passing he had worked these things out enough in his mind to have died in peace. Clara contemplated what new form his consciousness would have taken, for she believed in the evolution of creation through name and form and wondered how consciousness would again make itself useful.

Clara

After months of snow covering the ground, warmer weather came and, soon after, the first flowers appeared. Once the snow melted, these flowers—tiny, white, and bell-shaped, with large green leaves—pushed their way through the earth toward the sun. Clara compared Eli to those flowers and considered all of his guilt like the snow of a long winter season with many snowfalls, covering upon covering, making it difficult for spring to come, yet quiet and beautiful.

Similar to the snow was the dust on Clara's kitchen floor, how it quietly fell and created a covering, yet different from the snow in that the dust on her kitchen floor never really fell on dust in the way that snow falls on snow, because she swept daily. There was no real accumulation in the way that snow piles up after a long winter without any days warm enough for it to melt. She loved to sweep and it was actually this simple activity in the midst of her spiritual activities that uncovered for her the common ground.

All the qualities that she aspired to in her meditations were at work in her sweeping. While she made and picked up her piles of mostly crumbs and cat hair on the floor, the intention that she would remove layers of dirt accumulated in the storehouse of her mind always came to her. These thoughts were often nonverbal, but strong enough that she always felt better after sweeping. Sometimes she even scrubbed the floor of all past footsteps so cleanly that one could see oneself in the floor. But she knew that it could never stay like that. Someone would come, dropping a crumb or wearing shoes, so that while the pure ground could be reflected through the kitchen floor it had to exist within one's mental field, a clearing down to the finest level: so what was left belonged to everyone and was not individual or hers. Yet how could anyone experience this, when one's sense of individuality is so strong? How could this be shifted through sweeping?

Clara became philosophical, like many others who have to stay inside yet look out through many windows, outside at the snow and inside at the dust. These were times that brought about an introspection and analysis of her activities (at least the ones she repeated often) such that she would ask herself: *Why am I doing this? What is the hope behind these activities? What is the goal?* Questions like this often seemed unnecessary to her in that she looked upon her intentions as unfolding, changing, evolving, and mysterious. But especially on days of heavy snow, when she was indoors all day, it seemed a good opportunity to examine her intentions: otherwise there might be a purposelessness underlying her life.

During these times of reflection, she saw that most of her actions were not all good or all bad, but rather a mixture. She saw that mixed intentions lead to mixed results, and the forces of opposites, good and bad, were forces that she was living in the midst of. She saw that an honest look at everything would reveal this mixture and help her see the causes and consequences of her actions. This was a lot to take in, but she wanted to hold herself accountable, as she felt that otherwise her spiritual life would be compromised. The good that came from this was that it generated a lot of tolerance and forgiveness toward herself and others. As her mother Sarah always said, "People are not all black or white," as she felt that that was a simplistic vision of the world that was untrue. Of course, there are actions beyond categories, and these actions are free of any selfish intention or any sense of ownership, doer-ship, or desire for reward or acknowledgment. These types of actions are rare, but they do exist.

Theo

When Theo first became a nurse in New York City, the HIV/AIDS epidemic was at its height, and his first job was at St. Luke's Roosevelt on the night shift on what was called "the AIDS floor." Men, mostly in their twenties, thirties, and forties, were dying in large numbers, quickly. The virus they were dying of was highly contagious. Nurses were at risk because blood could carry the fatal disease from one person to another. Since they're always overworked, the floors are always understaffed, and the hours and shifts always long, nurses work to their edge and the edge is where accidents can happen. The nurses who worked on other floors didn't want to go near the AIDS floor; but since Theo was new to the job, he had no choice. As it turned out, many of the nurses on Theo's floor were men who had actually become nurses because of the HIV virus, because they sympathized with the men who were dying and wanted to be of help.

Since Theo worked the night shift, he saw a lot of what was called AIDS dementia, as this form of dementia is dominant in the nighttime. Patients would pull their IVs out, bleeding, and walk down the hallways, leaving blood all over the place and announcing that they were looking for some item—one that either didn't exist or existed but not in the hospital. Theo was alarmed and afraid at the sight of all this blood, knowing how infectious the disease was, but there were nurses whose first and every instinct was to take care of their patient. He saw them lovingly and physically bring these confused men back to their rooms, clean and comfort them, and put them back in bed. These actions weren't good or bad or mixed, because they were selfless.

But there are other selfless actions that are more common than being a nurse on the AIDS floor in the 1990s: like helping someone in the laundromat fold their sheets or helping someone fill out a complicated form or carry something heavy; holding the door open or simply stepping back and letting someone go ahead; or smiling at someone who is having a hard day. Clara once helped an elderly lady who had never been on an airplane buckle and unbuckle her seat belt, so that the lady felt safe. Of course, Clara didn't want anything in return. Just knowing that the lady felt safe was enough. Why was it that she so often forgot that this way of living less self-centeredly brought her happiness, as looking after one's self first gets so exhausting?

Clara

Clara often thought it would be helpful to examine the good and bad of her actions by writing a journal. She thought it would help her to see why she had done what she had done, and that the writing in and of itself would be an action that would help her to trace back her actions and reactions through the tunnels of her mind. She thought she would find residues or impressions left over from previous actions and that the knowledge of those imprints would allow her to understand herself and others better.

Once in a while she attempted to do this journal writing, but never got far. She would buy the journal, one whose look she liked, something she imagined good journal writing would be found in. She would open up to a blank page and think about her actions—whether she had managed her difficulties or could have acted with more care and awareness—but then would start daydreaming about Wise One: how at the end of his life, receiving one injection after another, he never complained; or how as a young man he had no money and couldn't even get a ticket for the free food at the canteen at the college.

Time would pass and if she ever got to writing it would be a poem about the landscape through the window, or she would stop writing and instead walk around the house cleaning the pictures that hung on her walls. Even without journal writing, she saw that many old ideas lingered in her and that if she put emphasis on them they would grow strong, and if she no longer found these ideas good or useful she could replace them with other ideas—but only if she knew in the first place that they were there, lingering.

After Wise One passed, Clara did not return to Sarana (the town in South India where Wise One and his family lived) for five years. This was a long time considering that for more than two decades she went once a year. When everyone asked why it had taken her so long to return, her mind went blank as if she herself did not know. But she did. Since she and Theo had moved from the city to somewhere remote and rural, far from other people—where time passes according to the motions of the sun, schedules are less insistent or important, and the weather (particularly the snowfalls and wind chills) are more extreme—it could get lonely by oneself.

Clara knew that this loneliness would be felt by her husband, and that the atmosphere of aloneness—not the "aloneness" of enlightenment, but rather of a man who misses his wife—would spread through the cabin and thicken the longer she was gone. He would not find soup on the stove or notes like *Be home by five, hope you had a great day* on the kitchen counter: So, not only would Theo miss Clara but the general peace and order felt in the house when she was there. Clara's traveling and time away had always been hard for Theo. Clara wondered whether in a previous life he'd been abandoned and if that abandonment, even if he was unconscious of it and it had occurred long ago, was influencing his desire for her not to leave home. Because of this, she decided that while she was in Sarana this time she'd write him letters daily. Theo came around to accepting the idea of her written offerings, and even said he would write back.

Clara was told she'd find Sarana very different than before, but she didn't find that to be so; in fact, for her nothing had really changed. There were more students from more countries and the prices of rickshaws, coconuts, or a plate of lemon rice had gone up, even doubled. There were more stray dogs. Other than that, life continued more or less the same, so that when she arrived and had her first meal at her favorite restaurant the waiter smiled in a spirit of recognition, remembering her and what she liked to order, and their conversation was more or less what it would have been five years previously.

In Sarana, routines and traditions were deeply ingrained in the lives of families. It seemed that these repetitive activities, especially those among women (cleaning, cooking, sewing, and all the responsibilities that came with managing a large family), had made these women strong and wise. Perhaps it was the way that service was built into their every waking moment or the wide range of skills they developed so that most women cooked every meal from scratch, made all the clothes, and cared for the children, the elderly, and/or a sick family member. While typically the men earned the money, the women were in charge of it, paid the bills, and knew how much things cost. While there is more to life than cooking and cleaning or providing for one's family, these women found a deep spiritual fulfillment in those daily activities very much in the way that sweeping satisfied Clara. It seemed to Clara that the Indian women, many still wearing saris, helped the children with their homework and the elders with their medicines, and kept everyone well-fed, while each day becoming kinder and closer to what lives on, in, through, and under all of creation.

Clara had her habits and routines, the ways in which she spent her time in Sarana, and though five years and Wise One had passed, in only a few days much was how it had always been. She went to the same restaurants to have breakfast and the same markets to buy fruits and crackers. She walked down the same busy streets with all the shops, or depending on her mood on the parallel streets that were residential and lined with trees and houses. When Clara looked up and saw the blue house with the pink front door and thought it was pretty, she remembered years ago looking up at the same pink house—*or was it the yellow one with the green door?*—and again thinking it was pretty, so that her memories and her present inclinations were embracing each other all the time.

She wondered how far back these memories would take her, feeling that possibly there was no end. Her recollections included feelings, like that of the ceiling fan above the bed turned on high; how she always wanted it on because she was hot, but was bothered by the way it blew a draft on her neck; or the feeling of the hour just before dawn and how she loved to meditate and study at that time.

So there she was after so many years, studying before sunrise under the ceiling fan, old and new Clara, and through these routines, patterns, and cycles, was relaxed. She too, like the Indian women around her that she so admired, accepted her routines and found within them many blessings. The Indian women had in the past frequently told her that actually she was Indian, only she'd been born abroad, and she believed this to be true.

She found that, in and out of the houses of the families who'd become her friends, teaching her over the years, not much had changed. Classes were still at five or eleven AM or 3:30 PM; periods for worship were still at six AM or seven PM; mealtimes were at eight AM, one PM, and again at nine in the evening, and still consisted mostly of rice. People rested during the hottest part of the day, which was from two to four. The women, even those such as Amala or Mira who taught, still had kitchen work that they were either busy with or that awaited them. Mira liked to say, "My work is waiting." Clara found the stability in these houses reassuring and considered these families fortunate. She knew there were those who hadn't had such experiences of stability and instead had had much restlessness or upheaval. They'd had to begin again in some new place, go to a new school, move into a new apartment, establish a new career, make new friends—sometimes more than once—and she thought that that would be difficult and perhaps perpetuate an outcome of continuous disappointment.

✼ ✼ ✼

Walking down the main street of Sarana, Clara passed a man with no legs she'd known from years before. His body was tied to a wooden platform with wheels on it and he pushed and pulled himself with the use of his arms. This man used to scare her and so she'd disliked and avoided him; until one day, to her relief, he no longer scared her and they became friends. Though they didn't speak the same language, they spoke to each other often. He appreciated and sensed her companionship and was happy about it, for Clara was not the only one who'd avoided him; many of the locals had as well. When Clara saw him, she remembered once disliking him and yet in the present moment he was her friend. She wondered what his life with no legs was like; what he would have had to work out, especially in his mind, to be capable of going on day in and day out, living in the streets year after year, in India. He recognized Clara and even smiled at her and in a small way she felt ashamed for all she had and took for granted.

She wondered if or when he would take a new birth, and whether this present hard life of his would facilitate or turn into the next life being something easier. She wondered if he had somehow chosen this life intentionally as a way of burning through old karmas quickly, or if the man without legs really had legs and just appeared legless to her because it was something that she needed to see. For all of these questions, she had no conclusions, for she knew that she knew nothing.

This man, whose name she never learned or even asked for, had over the years provoked many responses in Clara. At first fear, then a desire to avoid him. If she saw him, she went the other way, for looking at him was unpleasant and she turned away from unpleasant activities. Then he affected her emotionally and she could no longer pass him by. She saw him as a guru in disguise, a provider of lessons, a mirror to see herself in—one who inspired her kindness. Eventually, she bowed to him, and when she slipped him her monetary offering, it was with fruits, flowers, eye contact, and a genuine feeling of having looked forward to this encounter.

Perhaps all of her perceptions were mirrors, not just of this one man. For though it appeared that not much had changed in Sarana, the people seemed gentler and sweeter than she'd experienced before. This was true of the weather as well, so that even though it was in the high nineties, there were breezes and shady areas, and it grew cool at night. Though the population had actually increased, the town itself felt less crowded and polluted than in previous years, when she'd felt the congestion on the streets giving her anxiety. Even Clara's sense of herself had an ease to it: it was easy to wake up, to practice, to be among others or lie in bed reading, or sit still and concentrate for long periods of time. Where did all of this comfortableness, even with the man with no legs, come from? Clara wondered how much of what she experienced came from her own mind, or whether things were self-existent from their own side. Did the man with no legs exist if she did not know of him? Would his life be any less hard?

Clara had gone to the stand for a drink of coconut water when two young Indian women approached her, took her by the hands, and brought her inside a green house, where a few wooden tables were pushed up against each other in the middle of the front room. On the tables were plastic and glass necklaces and bracelets, hair ties and bobby pins, and sweets made from dates, cashews, chocolate, and rose petals. All the items were overpriced but the money was going to the Greenhouse, a shelter for women who'd been sold as children into brothels where they were forced to prostitute themselves and, later, having left the brothel were trying to live a more normal life. Clara knew about the organization from before because a friend of hers had stayed in the Greenhouse for several years, teaching the young women yoga to help them discover their self-worth. Despite the hardships that the girls had been through, they were proud of their jewelry. Clara chose a red-and-white beaded necklace.

An older woman in charge pointed out the girl who'd made it, who was happy with Clara's choice and smiling. The girl asked Clara her age and seemed surprised when Clara said fifty-three. Clara was accustomed to wearing the jewelry from her ancestors: rings and necklaces from her grandmothers and great aunts, or pocket watches and cufflinks from her grandfathers and uncles, that were later turned into broaches or earrings when they were handed down to their wives and daughters. These pieces were valuable, made from gold and decorated with precious stones. When Clara wore the jewelry, she knew her relations had worn it. The jewelry made by the girls, some of whom were prostitutes by the age of ten and were now twenty, was different in material worth and in their stories. But Clara valued the necklace she picked out and never forgot the smile on the girl's face and the question she asked about her age.

Clara wanted her letters to Theo to be special so in some way he'd be glad for her absence. She imagined him reading them with one of the cats on his lap, taking the letters to New York City when he visited Frances, reading them to her, and storing them in a drawer and rereading them years later. Behind all that she saw, heard, or thought, her ideas and impressions were the formations and substances of the paragraphs on blue stationary that she wrote to Theo while he was at home reading a book on the Jazz icons of America.

Dear Theo,

Today someone asked Mira what her name meant. She said Mira was the sea and that it was the name of one of Krishna's devotees who was also a princess. She said that in India the parents always named the children after the gods, but that that is now changing.

Yesterday I was walking through the downtown area of the city when a woman asking for money grabbed my skirt and would not let go. It scared me but I managed to calm her down and suggested we go for a tea or coffee. We went to Nalpak where the waiters all know me well. They let us sit for a long time even though the hours for lunch were over. On our short walk there I noticed she was limping and it seemed that one leg wasn't working. She told me that when she was four she was left on the doorstep of an orphanage. Above the front door of the orphanage was a sign that said LEAVE YOUR BABIES HERE INSTEAD OF KILLING THEM. She said that, thirty years later, the sign is still there.

When she was two she developed polio, which damaged her nervous system, so she could no longer use her right leg. Though the leg grew, she couldn't move it except by using her arms. She said she didn't feel sorry for herself; that she understood her parents were poor and igno-rant, and at that time it was difficult to get a polio vaccine. She said, "Wanting to free oneself of ignorance is a privilege my parents did not have." She was grateful they had not killed her.

Growing up in the orphanage she had a good disposition, was well liked, eventually got a basic education, and because she was good with numbers ended up with a job at a bank. This was against all odds as she had everything going against her: she was an orphan, woman, poor, handicapped, and ugly, for she said her disease had caused a deformity that stood out and that she was not well proportioned. Five years ago she had married a man who was also handicapped. As a young man he'd been working on a construction site when, in an effort to block the fall of someone else, he'd fallen from scaffolding. Recently, he'd been in a terrible accident when the fire from the cooking gas blew up in his face and his whole body was badly burned. She continued to tell me that his family never liked her because she came from a different caste. They blamed her for the fire and arrested her for attempted murder. She wasn't allowed to visit him in the hospital. Eventually, the claims against her were dropped, though many people still thought she was responsible—even people she'd thought of as her friends.

At this time she lost her good disposition, felt sorry for herself, and became destitute. Sitting on the sidewalk, her spirit broke and no one stopped to help her. She said I was the first person to talk to her in weeks.

When I told her I was from New York she said she knew of New York because that was where "the bomb blasts were": "9-11," she said. She wanted to know if I knew of anyone who died in the two buildings that had exploded and when I told her yes, I could tell by the compassionate and concerned way she looked at me that her good disposition was not completely gone. She said that she was so tired that she could sleep forever, even if it was on the sidewalk, and that she didn't mind anymore when people passed her by. She said that she had grown used to it so she wasn't sure why she had pulled on my skirt with such desperation except that somehow she knew I would help her.

After the tea we got into a rickshaw and went to Vidya and Rupa's orphanage. I thought she could stay there. She did not tell me her name. She said she changed her name when it was tied to the murder of her husband and so many false and mean things were said about the person with that name. "I am not that name," she kept saying. "Call me Nameless One." I thought that if she were to live at the orphanage, in time, when she was feeling better, she could work there in exchange for her stay. She said she used to be good with children, especially orphan children, who because of her own orphan background trusted her. They knew she was one of them.

When we were getting into the rickshaw, and Nameless One lifted her skirt in order to step up, I noticed her right leg, the one that didn't seem to be working, was a prosthetic made from plastic and mostly held together with duct tape. The leg was unsightly. I told her there was an expression back home "on your last legs" and that she should have the prosthetic leg fixed. She said it would be costly. The rickshaw driver turned to look at it. He said he had a friend who worked in plastics who could make a new one cheaply. She said she thought she was dreaming; that no one had cared about her or her leg for so long.

She seemed to like the ride out to the orphanage on the outskirts of town. It is less congested and there are many more trees, flowers, and birds within the coconut groves than in the downtown area. At the entrance to the orphanage above the gate is a sign, PAPAJI'S SCHOOL FOR CHILDREN. We both looked at the sign and then at each other. She was beautiful in a way: wild and tortured and poised. I forgot about everything and felt I was there entirely for her. She felt it and asked whether she could call me "Auntie Granny Sister." I said "Sister" would be fine. We got out of the rickshaw and together walked through the gate to a simple building made of cinder blocks, painted light blue with dark blue trim, with lots of potted plants all around and many of them flowering. Vidya and Rupa were sitting on the porch finishing their late lunch, for all the children eat before they do.

They were happy to see us and welcomed Nameless One. They asked the rickshaw driver to stay and join us for lunch, but he said he wanted to go see his friend who worked in plastics and asked to take another look at Nameless One's leg. Rupa got up and came back with a tape measure so the rickshaw driver could write down the exact size of the leg's height and width.

Soon afterwards we were served lunch. Rupa's cooking was always simple and nourishing and it tasted better than usual. Perhaps I was tasting it through my new friend, who was hungry for nourishment but also happiness, and Rupa's food contained both. Again Nameless One said she thought she was dreaming: that she was afraid she would wake up and be back on the sidewalk in the downtown area. As I told Rupa and Vidya Nameless One's story, she confirmed she had not caused the cooking gas to explode. She loved her husband, they had had a good marriage; she'd always wanted to be with someone handicapped, as disadvantaged people know the world differently and have a wisdom that comes with or through their disabilities.

Vidya and Rupa listened with care and kindness. They said they couldn't call Nameless One by that name, and asked her if she liked the name Atithi Devo. They explained that Atithi was Sanskrit for guest, that Atithi Devo referred to the guest as God, and that in ancient times when communication was not as easy as it is today no one knew when

FELL IN HER HANDS

guests would be arriving. Vidya said that because travel before modern times had a lot of hardship and there weren't as many hotels or lodges as there are today, people would stop for food and lodging wherever they could find them; often at other people's homes. It says in the scriptures, which Vidya was already reciting, that the unannounced guest and God were the same because God arrived unexpectedly. Like that, Nameless One accepted the name of Atithi Devo and said she'd never call or think of herself as Nameless One again.

While Vidya was reciting from the scriptures, Atithi Devo noticed the picture of Ramakrishna hanging above the front door. She knew Ramakrishna was one of India's saints from the last century and that he taught that there was no greater form of worship than to take care of others. Eventually, some details were discussed. Vidya and Rupa asked Atithi Devo what her skills were. She said she'd lost her skills. They said her skills would come back, that she needed rest, and that being with the children would do her good.

After lunch, we walked across the field to several small huts made from mud and grass. We went inside one of them. It was plain and clean, and furnished with a bed, a chair, a dresser, and another picture of Ramakrishna. Vidya and Rupa said to Atithi that this would be her room, that they'd bring her a bucket of water so she could bathe, and that they'd bring her clean clothes. They told her not to worry, that everything would be OK. She turned and in a low voice said to me that she was hesitant to believe them: her disappointments were so large, her trust in others so shaken . . . and yet they were persuasive.

I left her there and Vidya took me back in his truck to where I was staying.

Vidya said we would have to wait to see how deep her wounds were: whether or not she would get along with the others; whether or not she would want to change. He reminded me that life there was basic, without luxuries, not even running water or electricity. They burn candles for light, sleep on the floor, eat porridge . . . pull the water up from the well in buckets, carry it to the kitchen, and pour it into vessels for cooking, drinking, and washing. They bathe with cold water even in the cooler months. Of course, he said that all this was better than to live on the sidewalk and that mainly through the blessings of Ramakrishna their lives were made comfortable. "Yes," he kept saying, "we will have to wait and see."

I thanked him, bowed to him in a gesture of respect, touched his feet, and told him that I would stop by soon. He said he would look after Atithi and that she was in the hands of Ramakrishna now. He blessed me and said it had been nice to see me. I came inside and immediately started writing this letter.

Love, Clara

Theo read the letter while standing in the middle of the road. He'd opened it up by the mailbox. He hadn't intended to read the letter there, but found himself so engaged after the first sentence that he couldn't stop reading nor move to another place. When he was finished, he folded the letter up, put it in his pocket, walked down the driveway, through the field, into the house, and sat down on the daybed completely transported by his wife's letter. He wondered what the chances were that Clara had chosen to walk down the road where Nameless One was sitting in desperation on the sidewalk. He questioned why it had been *her* skirt that the poor woman pulled on so urgently instead of another's. Was this destiny, interdependence, fate, *karma*, God? Who was in charge and why was it that Clara often seemed to be at the right place at the right time to be instrumental?

Dear Clara,

Last week I rented a wheelchair for Frances and took her to the park to see the cherry blossoms. The chair costs five dollars a day and if I decide I want to buy it they will deduct whatever money I'd spent renting it. At first, she didn't want to go to the park and wanted only to buy food. She is so used to thinking only in terms of her survival when it comes to what she needs from outside her apartment. But later she asked if I wanted a coffee and since I don't drink coffee I said no, but now I regret it as I realize it was probably her way of asking for one for herself. Her desires are so small yet all the time they are accompanied by the feeling that they will not be fulfilled. When we got home, she was so tired she slept until the next day; but upon waking she was ready to talk about Albert Camus' The Myth of Sisyphus and the symbolism of pushing the rock up the mountain.

Before I left to visit Frances, I had a patient whom I used to know when I lived on the Lower East Side. I didn't really know her but I saw her all the time riding her bicycle, even in the rain. I recognized her as I was taking down her family history. She told me that as a child she traveled a lot with her father who was a clown in a medium-sized circus. When she was fifteen, she fell off a trapeze and dislocated her hip. She wasn't supposed to be on it but she was always watching the trapeze artists and it looked like fun, like they were flying. So one day she thought she would try. After that, she had to have a hip replacement and since then never felt healthy. In her adult life she became a writer. She has published four books and has a new book coming out in a few weeks time, though she may not live that long. She says that people like her books and that when she rides her bike through the streets of NYC people call out to her, "Hey you're Martha . . . loved your last book!" As she was telling me all this I thought of how little we know of people we see all the time, like in the streets or at the grocery store.

Anyway, a week ago, while visiting a friend who lives not too far from us, she had a heart attack. She said she wasn't feeling different than usual nor was she upset about anything. She's only fifty and is now hooked up to various life-support machines. Today, when I arrived at work she was unconscious.

Apparently, she has been that way for the last three days and since I've had the last four days off and was in NYC I did not know this. I was thinking I would ask her about The Myth of Sisyphus, *but she is dying and her body is breaking down. As the word of her heart attack is spreading, I have the feeling the whole world is praying for her. I can't explain it. It's hard being a nurse. When someone dies, even though I had the last four days off, I feel responsible.*

Love, Theo

Clara read Theo's letter and contemplated writing back. It had been a weeklong holiday in India and all of her classes had been canceled. She had spent the week eating out and taking pictures of dogs. Restaurant food in India is tasty and inexpensive. Nalpak, Clara's favorite restaurant, always had a daily special and she knew them by heart, so that even when she was at home in her cabin in the woods, far away from Nalpak, she thought to herself what day it was and linked it to the daily special. Monday was ragi roti; Tuesday, deep-fried rava idly; Wednesday, banana bhaji; Thursday, garlic noodles with chili; Friday, tomato dosa; Saturday, lemon rice; and Sunday, potato balls. Year after year, these specials and the day in which they were served would never change.

Restaurants are lively and crowded and often if one goes alone, you'll end up sitting at a table with others. Sometimes, Clara likes to order a dish simply because of its name, like ammalaki upma, and since she only goes to vegetarian restaurants, she doesn't have to worry that she will find chicken bones or other forms of animals in the food. Even if the order is something plain, it always comes with a curry, chutney, or pickle. As soon as one is finished eating, someone comes to clear and clean the table. It used to be children, who were barefoot and looked hungry, and this would bother Clara to such an extent that she'd feel sick. But nowadays laws have been put into place, and it's mostly elderly women who pick up the plates and wipe down the tables, and for the most part they appear happy and healthy as well.

Since classes were canceled Clara felt it was OK to eat more than usual, but at the same time she was thinking of the porridge that the workers and residents at the orphanage ate and that they didn't have daily specials there or in many other places. She also thought that the austerities around food that saints and sadhus or pilgrims adhered to were probably necessary to commune with a higher force and that oatmeal and broth would eventually be the food she lived on. But she was not yet at that point of letting go, especially when in India, where Nalpak was serving such delicious food.

Dear Theo,

All I do lately is eat the daily special at Nalpak and photograph the stray dogs living in the city. Some of them I think I recognize from previous years. I see that over time they get damaged from street life, just as humans do. I don't think any of them have ever had an "owner," so you can't really call them stray because they haven't strayed from anywhere. People call them "menaces," "nuisances," "stupid," and "dirty," but the truth is the dogs keep themselves clean most of the time. It is only when they are beaten or go hungry that they stop grooming themselves, also like humans. That's why the children in the streets eventually become dirty . . . not because they are "dirty" but because of their hunger. Look at any child whose clothes smell and hair is matted, and they will be hungry.

People say that the dogs bite, but they only do so when provoked. People say the dogs make a mess out of the garbage but if there weren't so much garbage in the first place the dogs wouldn't make a mess of it. People who ride bikes say the dogs chase them so they throw stones at the dogs to get them to stop. Why not feed them instead? In front of the dogs people say, "We should send them to China where people eat dog. . . ." It's terrible. Once in a while, someone will hit a dog to death with a stick more or less for sport. The dogs' threshold for pain is high. Their lives are hard. They're not much cared for. They look after each other, like children without parents, the oldest one taking charge. If they are hanging out and not rushing down the street I will take their picture. I have made many dog friends since arriving here. They don't want for anything in exchange for their picture but I always offer food, which they receive graciously. They are not spoiled. They don't know that dogs in other places live in houses with families where someone cooks for them, they sleep on beds, they are given fancy names like Valentino or Chardonnay, and are groomed and loved by their owners.

Eating the daily specials and taking pictures of the dogs is enough for me.

I don't feel that I am missing out on anything although I know that others are putting their time to better use. I am not harming anyone and I don't overeat. The photographs speak in wordless ways without dog- or people-language. Did you ever read The Stray Dog? *It's about a man who is having a mental breakdown and mistakes himself for a dog who is treated so badly that he mistakes himself for garbage. But I haven't read it and I could have the story all wrong.*

Clara

Clara was referring to a short story written by Sadeq Hedayat, an Iranian writer who committed suicide in 1951 at the age of forty-eight. Theo had not read *The Stray Dog*, although he did know something about it and although he didn't think Clara's description was accurate, he liked it nonetheless. That is the beauty of interpretations and perceptions; they are influenced by the mood of the mind of the one interpreting, and will always be personal.

Dear Clara,

As I sit to write, looking out of the windows, I see a wild turkey moving with grace and care across our field. I can just hear you saying, "It's terrible that people eat turkeys. Hopefully the animal will stay here where he or she won't be killed." The bird's feathers are arranged on top of its head in a way that determines the sex of the bird, but I can't remember if the feathers on top mean the bird is male or female. A black crow is here also. The bird came near the front door where the little bird has returned to her nest in the cross beams of the overhang where most certainly she has laid eggs. I worried the crow, hungry for the little bird's eggs, would destroy the nest, so I shooed the crow away. But I can't guard the nest all day.

Spring came fast and already there are ants and bees inside the house. Ling got stung yesterday when a yellow jacket was on the kitchen towel she picked up off her kitchen counter. The sting is really painful and the itching lasts for days. Meanwhile, the screen on the upstairs window is not properly in place but every time I remember that it needs fixing I've already had a glass of wine and it's starting to get dark. I don't think it's a good idea to get up on a ladder if I'm tipsy. As I write all of this I think to myself how unromantic I've become. But it's not unromantic. It's the house, land, windows, screens, and bees that surround our love and life in the hum of springtime.

As always, Theo

Gita

It has been many years since Clara and Gita first met. Clara remembers her first lessons in the family house in Sarana well. That house belonged to Mr. Chandra's student, who had moved to California and was letting Mr. Chandra and his family live there rather than renting it to tenants. His job in California paid enough money that he could afford to do what he wanted with the house in Sarana, and he loved the Chandra family. But eventually he came back and the family had to move out. It was at that time, when Gita was twenty-four, that Mr. Chandra lost his job.

After Gita's family left Sarana, they lived in a slum in Bangalore. The apartment wasn't too uncomfortable and her mother kept it clean, but the buildings in that part of the city were so close to each other that no one had any privacy or quiet. The infrastructure had not developed as fast as the construction of new buildings or the population growth so there was always the problem of garbage, sewage, and noise.

Gita was getting her Master's Degree in Engineering from the local college. She was offered many scholarships from the best schools throughout India but decided to accept the one that came from the nearest school, though not the best, so that she could remain at home and look after Anjali, her blind younger sister, who is also an extraordinary singer. The nerve that sends messages from Anjali's retina to her brain does not work. It is a rare disease that does not cause her pain, but she needs constant care. She can see shapes and make her way around her home, but anywhere else she needs escorting. She did not learn braille as a child because her family thought it would prevent her from using the little sight that she has. Mr. and Mrs. Chandra have always wondered whether that was a mistake. They are anxious that Gita gets married. They think she is waiting to finish her degree, but in truth she is afraid that if she gets married she will be abandoning her sister, who needs her support, but Gita has never mentioned this to her parents.

Their neighbor carries stones from one pile to another. He works on a construction site where the boss is so stingy that, rather than buy a wagon to load and move the stones, he pays the young man almost nothing to move them. Stone men in India are low on the ladder of the caste system and it's possible that the stone man's boss enjoys watching the man toil and break his back in exchange for unfair wages. The stone man has broad shoulders and narrow hips and tilts his head to one side. Something about the way he stands still and leans forward, as if into the wind or some other invisible support, would make one think he's injured or in pain or has experienced one (or perhaps more than one) tragedy. But he never talks about himself in that way. In the evenings he sits in front of his door in the hopes that Gita may pass by. If she is carrying potatoes, rice, books, or flowers, he will help her. He would like to marry her but does not think she will want to marry a stone man.

When Clara first studied with Mr. Chandra she wanted a lesson every day. Even if he were busy, she would convince him to give her a short lesson by saying, "What if I come for ten minutes and you could teach me something small?" He knew she treasured her time with him. He said, "Even though she is Western, she has advanced quicker than most of my students whose parents force them to come. Her devotion is great." He said that devotion keeps one learning. He'd say, "Without devotion, nothing can be learned, because you won't stick with something long enough."

When Clara arrived in Bangalore and saw the squalor that surrounded the apartment of the Chandra family, it greatly unsettled her. The activity on the streets, even as you walked into their building, was threatening and unwelcoming, and an undercurrent of crime pervaded. She wanted to avoid eye contact or contact of any sort with anyone and get into the apartment quickly. Once in the apartment, she could see that Gita's mother had changed. She looked worn, tired, and frightened; Clara gathered it was on account of the new living quarters.

Gita was delighted to see Clara, and the two of them immediately began catching up on each other's lives. Gita shared her reason for not wanting to get married. She said that with her help Anjali had scored ninety-eight percent on her exams. Clara said, "Someone will want to marry you that will also want to look after Anjali, who will appreciate Anjali and your love and devotion to your sister; someone who will enjoy hearing the two of you singing together, and feel doubly blessed to have you and your sister in their life. You're a beautiful, mature, simple woman. You will make a wonderful wife to some lucky and well-deserving man. You will see . . . it's wonderful to be married." Gita seemed like she had the same hopes as well, but Indian people, or poor people, are sometimes afraid to hope.

Clara

Before Clara left for Sarana, Marigold's husband gave her an expensive cell phone to use on her trip. He'd given such phones to everyone in his family and had what was called a "family plan" that included Clara. In this way, she never paid any monthly charges for her phone. The phone was small, she could put it in her pocket, though it was not advised since it was electronic and would not be good to keep close to her skin. Within the phone was a camera and the camera had a feature where she could point the lens back at herself.

One night, Clara walked to the small house where men and women sit together to sing to the picture of their guru. This was the house where she had spent many happy evenings. When the singing was over, Clara joined the line of people making their way down the stairs and out through the front gate. Just before the gate were two ladies, one handing out cookies and the other flowers. Clara put the flowers in her hair, which was longer than it had been in years, and ate the cookies while she walked home. When she got into her room, she was happy from the evening and felt like taking her picture and sending it to Theo. She was wearing white and had a glow about her. By lightly touching a few buttons on her phone, placing her finger on certain symbols—one of a camera, the other of an envelope—the picture of herself was taken and sent all the way back to Theo in their cabin in upstate New York. That was the sequence of events. She had gone to the singing; come back elated; had the idea to take her picture, which she took and sent to Theo; who within a few hours opened the email and saw the picture by clicking on the symbol of a paperclip, which stood for an attachment.

Theo looked at the picture of his wife sideways, for he couldn't figure out how to rotate the picture right-side-up, but nonetheless was struck by how lovely his wife looked. It was true that Clara always looked exceptionally well in Sarana, surrounded by her teachers and spending most evenings wearing white and singing. Theo sent an email back to Clara telling her that she looked beautiful. Though Theo was not the only one to compliment her on her looks, somehow it mattered most to her how he saw her, such that his praise after twenty years of marriage made her feel beautiful in a way that nothing else could. It was through his eyes that she wanted to look beautiful. He was like a light, casting beauty upon her through the perceptions of his mind. Clara's mood was enhanced by his message. She thought of the stained glass she'd seen in churches in Europe and the rays of sunlight colored by passing through the glass, and she compared his vision of herself to the windows.

Bena

Clara traveled from Sarana to Madu with her Sanskrit teachers, Amala and her brother Neelambar. It was the one-year anniversary of the death of Amala's husband's mother, and because of that they did not want to eat food prepared outside of their home even though the trip took over fifteen hours. Amala had woken up extra early and prepared food for the three of them, so that midway through the trip they pulled off the highway, onto the "nice" road, and "cut a left," parked under a tree, and had their lunch. This meal of semolina with peanuts and mustard seeds—carefully packed with bowls, spoons, lime pickles, chutney powder, and drinking water— touched Clara, and she did not perceive it as an ordinary lunch. Nothing was ordinary when she was with her teachers, and she wanted to have this mindset of appreciating everything more often. Was this what it was to be in the presence of the Divine? If so, isn't this what she wanted all along? These were the questions she pondered on her way to Madu.

In Madu, the three of them went to the ashram of the saint affectionately called Sri Rama. It was there that they met Bena. Clara had known of Bena through Stella, an old and dear friend whom she referred to as her spiritual sister. Stella had told Clara to visit Bena if she was ever in Madu, and that Bena was a great storyteller. Bena would welcome her visit since she was a friend of Stella's, because Bena thought Stella was an angel, a holy being, an emanation of a feminine side of Sri Rama, so that even though Bena was in her nineties and not receiving visitors, she'd make a special exception for Clara or anyone who was a friend of Stella's.

When they arrived and Bena came to the door, Clara knew that this would be one of those rare visits you have with someone that comes as an unexplained gift, sign, marker, or symbol—as if being on a trail and following the red or blue circles to the mountaintop. As soon as Bena began talking, Clara asked if she could record the visit so she could send the recording to Stella, and Bena agreed that it would be OK. Before sending the recording to Stella, Clara played it once for herself. At first it was just to check on the sound quality of the recording, but then she became engrossed in Bena's story:

> At one point, I don't remember when, my name became Bena, Bena means "elder sister." Though I have no blood sisters, I am the oldest in my community and have been living in the ashram since the early days. Many of the elders from my generation have passed, and since I am

an elder to the younger generation, I got the name Bena. Also, I never married nor was involved romantically with anyone, and "elder sister" also means Sister or nun. Many foreigners come to visit me, especially since I spent time with Sri Rama, and for people outside of my country, Bena is an easy name to remember and pronounce.

When I was young, my parents wanted me to marry, but I knew from an early age I was different. I wanted to be free of the responsibilities of family life so I could focus completely on God. I was never tempted to live a worldly life. My father was an engineer and built bridges over turbulent waters and for that we traveled a lot. I met Sri Rama when I was seventeen; at once, it was strange and familiar. I felt he had the divine spark in him and I was happy to be in his atmosphere. I went to live with him, and at that time a small community of followers and friends, in the forest. Though I left my family to be with him, my association with Sri Rama benefited everyone close to me: my parents, siblings, grandparents, aunts, uncles, and cousins. At every step, Sri Rama's helping hand was there, protecting them.

At one point in my life, I traveled a lot. This was after Sri Rama passed and more people around the world wanted to know what he was like. A small group of us, led by Pandit-ji, went all over Europe and America. There, I saw many devotees and I realized that his impact had spread far.

As I grew old, I had a maternal instinct toward the younger generation, so although I never had children I experienced a strong motherly feeling. In a previous life I am sure I experienced motherhood.

Living in the ashram was like living in the presence of the Divine. Sri Rama was not an ordinary human, and to be close to him and in his proximity over time I became in some small way like him. The ashram was a branch of heaven on Earth's soil. In its first days, we were a small community, a family really. Sri Rama encouraged us to be "all-rounders," and put us through everything. We learned music, dance, and painting, performed plays, and read and wrote poetry. The intensity of the arts was part of our spiritual training. Everything was so informal. There was joy in the air. As the ashram grew and more people were visiting, rules and regulations had to be put into place. The formalities and the large numbers of people did not affect Sri Rama's meditations in that, as it had always been, whenever he would sit and go into deep meditation, all the birds, butterflies, and animals who lived in the surrounding woods would come to be near him. Through Sri Rama we learned to love animals and that the best way to see them is when they are free.

Two years ago, I thought I was having my final hour, my last breath. But somehow, I passed through it. Since then, I realized I am many people. I only appear as one, because I am encased in a body. This became clear to me, as suddenly a veil was lifted before my eyes. I saw that no one comes to the ashram; we are all brought here. My consciousness crossed a boundary, and I often feel I don't exist. Since then, I am more in my subtle body. It is not solid or concrete.

Because of this, even if I am sick, I look well. I always look well. People frequently comment on my healthy looks and yet I know I am fading. I visualize and approach, without struggle, my peaceful death. . . .

At that point, the tape recorder stopped working. It was as if fate intervened, so that her words would remain unrecorded.

Clara

Clara was in the central railway station in Chennai, India. It was four AM, and the station was crowded for that time of morning, but quiet. She was traveling back to Sarana from Madu. Her train was at six AM. She had traveled through the night by car. She was afraid the driver would fall asleep while driving or that the car would break down. She was afraid that if she got to the station too early, it might be dangerous to have to pass time there in the middle of the night. She was also afraid that if she got there late she'd miss the train. Train reservations are hard to get and this particular booking was made weeks in advance. She was sitting in the railway station's waiting room, for which she had to pay thirty rupees (the equivalent of fifty cents), and show her railway ticket. Outside the waiting room people were sleeping anywhere and everywhere, spread out on the floor amongst their luggage. It was dirty and mosquitoes were buzzing around, but because of the hour the atmosphere was calm.

The waiting room was mostly for women who were traveling either alone or with other women. It felt safe in the waiting room. The bathroom was clean and Clara washed her face and hands and was happy to be in the waiting room. She was alone in that she didn't have a traveling companion, but she didn't feel lonely. Two men were in charge of the waiting room. They were wearing brown-colored uniforms and sat at a small table by the entrance door. One collected the money and the other distributed the "railway waiting-room ticket." The thirty rupees separated mostly first-class travelers from the rest. In India, small amounts of money served as fees that kept people of different financial backgrounds in different waiting rooms. Even the highways were like this because only the drivers who could afford the highway permit were allowed on the highway. This kept the majority of the traffic off the highway, especially the slower vehicles. Everywhere in the world such divisions are made. Human beings divide.

Sitting in the waiting room, Clara didn't feel separate from the others. Everyone, including Clara, wanted to wash their face and hands in the bathroom and keep their personal belongings nearby. Everyone was tired as it was the middle of the night. Everyone had their story, a place to go, and a reason why. If anyone needed help, one of the men in uniform would help. They had looked at Clara's ticket and would make sure she got on her train; even if she fell asleep they would wake her. That would be seen as their duty. They took their job seriously.

Clara had traveled to India wanting to better understand herself and others. She felt that kind of inner journey would happen easier there. The Eastern philosophies gave a context to her experiences. The emphasis on consciousness as truth and love, as an unlimited network shared by all of creation, is deep-rooted in Indian people. This way of viewing the world is comfortable to her. She spent a lot of time in nature watching plants grow. If a seed was put in soil, in two to three days it sprouted because consciousness was there. If she was there to see it sprout, her consciousness saw the consciousness of the seed and the soil. If she wasn't there, whether the seed still sprouted or the soil still was nourishing was of interest to her.

Philosophies get interpreted differently by people at various places and times, according to circumstance, influence, background, upbringing, culture, education, language, religion, geographic location, etc. What interested Clara about philosophy was how it could be utilized to better the world. Only then, did it become relevant for her. Because of her work as a teacher, she had done a lot of traveling around the world. One concern she had wherever she went was how the animals were treated. It seemed that wherever she went, animals were abused. They were seen as put on Earth for the benefit of humans, to use however humans like, but with no purpose of their own. Even plants were viewed like that, here to beautify the world for humans but not for their own life. If one desired to chop down a tree or a plant in order to have a better view, no one thought anything of it. If one cut the limb off an animal, depending on which animal, it might have been considered more serious than a branch on a tree, but only when it was a human limb was it really considered harmful.

This was because the all-pervasiveness of consciousness was seen by only a few rare souls. Clara desired to be one of these souls and at times felt herself moving in that direction as if water flowing from a higher to a lower land: happening without her efforts, naturally going toward her goal, no longer a need for discipline. She always had the feeling that of all the people she knew who wanted to reach enlightenment, Sun would reach this goal and take Clara along with her. She knew that Sun had lost interest in purchasing material objects other than what she required, for more than that she would consider excess. She knew that Sun did not use up any mental energy over such things, that in terms of the material world what she carried was light, and in this way she would swim across the ocean of worldly miseries and reach her final destination of freedom soon.

As her last day in India was approaching, Clara couldn't help but be mentally carried back to America. What she missed most, of course, was Theo. In Sarana, her studies centered on understanding the existence of various states or levels of consciousness. These levels, each one subtler than the previous, were goals for the serious student to move toward. But the movements, though she herself had traveled a great distance from her home, were not external: they were internal—one was moving toward one's Self. But traveling to distant lands always helped Clara to travel within herself and to feel a part of her that would otherwise remain dormant. She herself had not been able to maintain states of total desirelessness for long, but through her studies she did have an intellectual understanding of them and this helped her manage the ups and downs of her life gracefully. She understood that no matter how abstract or esoteric the teachings became, no matter how layered, the basic concept of getting along with others could never be discarded.

The family in Sarana that Clara stayed with were not Brahmins and not religious. The old man owned a men's clothing shop downtown. His son had taken it over and his grandson would be working there when he finished school. His wife was the head of the household and managed all the cooking and cleaning. Since all the family's meals were eaten at home, and the men refused to eat leftovers, she and her daughter worked all the time. Her daughter had two young children whom she helped to do everything, from getting dressed to understanding and finishing their homework. After lunch the whole family rested, spread out on couches, with a small TV going in the background, though no one seemed too interested in it.

Like all families, especially when three generations live in one household, arguments occurred, but in this family they quickly passed, with no animosity and grudges, and soon everyone would be getting along again. Even at the height of yelling the atmosphere was loving. They could never remain mad at each other, and they would be laughing soon after an argument. They got along and loved each other. "Otherwise," one of them would say, "why else should we be living together?" There was nothing separate or hidden. What Clara saw—the cooking, cleaning, resting, quarreling, and making up, the meals together, the sharing of extremes in weather (hot in summer when the sun was piercing, damp and wet during the monsoon when the rains were heavy) was what it was: their life. Over the many years that Clara stayed there, this underlying harmony, what she thought of as the soul of the family, never changed. The family was stable and this firmness of the family, in a household where water and electricity came and went, was a great support for her evolution, so that she never wanted to stay anywhere else when she was in Sarana.

Eli

My name is Eli, but Lothar, Kurt, Ernest, Albert, or Max are names that in subtle ways, for sentimental reasons, I also identify with. Since I am no longer in a physical body as I was as Eli I no longer need a single name. I was hoping my daughter Clara would have named her children Ernest, Max, Lothar, or Albert. Even if she'd had girls, she could have called them Ernestine, Maxine, Charlotte, or Alberta. But she didn't have children.

In November of 2009, my heart stopped beating in the middle of the night and my soul exited from the body it had entered so many years before. This occurred while I was sleeping under the afghan that was given to me by the nurses at the hospice center. I don't know if they were actually nurses but they were certainly caregivers. There was one woman I remember well who sat with me for many hours in the last four days of my life. Sarah was too old and tired to sit with me for those final hours, but after fifty-three years of marriage it was not necessary. We had already exchanged a few apologies and some tender words of immense gratitude and that had been enough to end our physical life together.

Sarah kept the afghan. She likes it because it gives her a feeling of contact with me. It was one of the last few possessions. She remembers it covering my legs, for I was thin and cold and was hardly eating by the time I was wrapping my legs with knitted blankets.

A few days after my enlarged heart stopped beating, the body was buried. Men whom I had not known dug a hole, lowered the simple casket that contained the body into the hole, and filled the hole back up with the soil and sub-soil that they'd removed through the digging of the hole. Mixed in with the earth were small rocks, sand particles, dried leaves, insects, and worms.

Meanwhile, the rabbi said a few consoling words and traditional prayers to those who were huddled around the casket placed within the hollow at the grave site.

After everyone left, the flesh and bones began rotting and sinking into the ground. Had I been standing, the weight would have dropped down into the feet and the hands would have remained empty. But the body was reclining, decaying, horizontal, and relieved, expanding and neutral, while I was witnessing from below and above in a state of complete equilibrium the goodness of my life. Suspended beneath the world, I was surprised by how easy it was to let go.

This was the peace Clara had wanted for me when I was still alive.

I would be sitting in the deep red chair in my slippers with swollen ankles, constipation, chest pain, and thoughts of life, some happy but mostly not, when Clara would say, "Dad, please think positively. Your final thoughts will set the tone for your next life." But at that time I had the feeling there would not be a "next life" as Clara put it, but rather just flesh and bones being eaten by worms and insects. I would continue to exist inside of those worms and insects and the other animals that would eat the worms and insects that had eaten me. That food chain would be the "next life" for me. I wondered how with all my human-acquired knowledge I would taste to an animal that had not formally studied as I had. Would I, buried in the ground, parallel to bridges and perpendicular to trees, unlearn what I had learned? Would the understandings of my past experiences break apart, fade away, decompose, and turn into seeds that would ripen and grow as grass on a field of science somewhere, anywhere, elsewhere, possibly, probably, in Europe?

But as it is, pairs of opposites, even life and death, in this dust realm unite and resolve in a merger. For it is the trees in the cemetery that grow (some six stories high, others wide and broad that like the roof of a house serve as a protective covering), that flower every spring and attract so many birds, butterflies, insects, and other forms of life amongst the tombstones and bones beneath—that prove (as a scientist will always need proof) that life and death are one. But I never said these things to Clara. Instead I said, "You're probably right. . . . I should think more positively," as I was too old and tired to speak about the "after life" or next life with my daughter.

Sarah

In one way I outlived my husband and in another way I have not. He is absent and present. He is present in my thoughts in the form of memories, which is funny because I can't remember anything about the day: what I did; what I ate (if I ate); what time I woke up; what book I'm reading (if I'm reading); whether the children called or are visiting; if

I've gone to the store, picked up the mail, read the newspaper, or even bathed. Yet I clearly remember Eli's way of interlacing his fingers and setting his hands on the table or the sound of him in his slippers shuffling around the kitchen.

I suppose after more than fifty years of marriage Eli will always be in my thoughts wandering through my mind as if it was his own, without any barriers preventing him from keeping me company, especially in the evenings when the activities of the day have ceased.

I feel his presence in many of the things in the apartment: the books, the rugs, his mother's china, the old red chair. I feel his absence in the bedroom in that there's only one bed now instead of the two twin beds pushed up against each other. And when I open the refrigerator I don't see broccoli or prunes.

There's a lot of Eli in the children and grandchildren, especially in my daughter Clara, who has his eyes and a fair amount of his temperament—especially when she's arguing a point, in the way that even if it's illogical she can be persuasive.

In a strange way, he is present in my evening glass of wine because he never drank alcohol and therefore I never did either except on special occasions, like weddings or parties, which became more rare as we aged. So in the evenings, when I pour myself a glass of wine, I always think of him and how we never drank. We also never shared clothes. He never went into my closet and most of the time I don't think he even noticed what I was wearing, although had I ever been really un-presentable he would have noticed. Clara complains that her husband wears her clothes all the time, but that would never have happened with Eli. Eli liked reading the New York Times. He said that our subscription caused suspicion in our neighbors during the years that we lived in Southern California. He liked Tuesday's edition for science and Sunday's for the travel section.

I recently had what Dr. O'Day called a minor heart attack. He just came in the room and said, "You've had a heart attack," and then he left. That was it. He didn't ask how I was feeling or if I was up for a little chat, or whether I liked the hospital food, or any of the questions that would have brought the humanity up a level. He got to things quickly: head on, with no time to go slowly about such matters. But he did take good care of me, and after three days I was discharged and feeling much better. The children came to pick me up and it happened to be my birthday. When I saw them coming through the doorway of my room announcing that they were there to "take me away," "Happy Birthday" it was indeed.

When the orderly came with the discharge papers there were no explanations of results from the numerous tests I had incurred during my stay at the hospital, so that I left a little *unsure of how well or worn out my eighty-eight-year-old heart actually was. Clara was upset by this lack of closure and remembers a hospital discharge as something more formal, with more papers to sign and a final visit from the doctor. Then the doctor would say, "Do you have any questions?" such that even if that visit was short a lot would be accomplished. But the doctor did not come and we basically just walked out.*

In the evening, after having a long and wonderful bath, Theo and I spoke at length about Ibsen and Strindberg. I prefer Hedda Gabler, *he prefers* Miss Julie. *I found that even after a small heart attack Ibsen is still important and that in our discussion I could for the most part find the words I was looking for.*

❈ ❈ ❈

On the night of Sarah's birthday and discharge from the hospital, Clara, having not read Ibsen or Strindberg in a long time, and not having a memory anything like her husband's or her mother's for the plays and novels she had read, still enjoyed the conversation. She was used to listening to the two of them speak of the books they had read, remembered, and interpreted differently. These conversations were stories in and of themselves that described a vast range of experiences—including dreams, suicides, insanity, secrets, and a full spectrum of financial circumstances. Each story somehow seemed part of the next and Clara reflected on her own story while the events or nonevents of these written stories were being spoken of.

Sarah thought it was the small events in life and in books that were interesting, like the way someone with a headache would rest their head on a pillow; while Theo was more interested in bigger events like death, murder, or revolution. When "the children" were leaving, Clara encouraged Sarah to rest at least for a few days and to consider her heart attack seriously.

Sarah responded with a light-hearted "I'm not afraid to die," but Clara explained that it wasn't death she was afraid of either, but something worse, like a stroke, where her mother would not be able to find the words she was looking for.

Emmet

Last year in the beginning of summer, I visited my friend Clara. It was blueberry season and she had made a pie with the intention of photographing the pie and then afterwards she, my girlfriend, her husband, and I could eat it. The pie was delicious and Clara said several times that there was no milk, eggs, or butter in the pie such that no animals had been enslaved for our pleasure. I could tell from its texture, taste, and weight, as well as Clara's description of the pie, what the pie looked like. Later that evening she showed and explained to us the photos she had taken of the pie. She said the pie was placed on an old wooden table in an almost-empty room, with nothing new or fancy in it. I knew the pictures were beautiful. I knew that Clara could photograph a pie and in one picture communicate varying meanings, making the viewer work hard to see themselves in the picture they were looking at, causing one to reflect and take note of one's life, often fraught with distractions and hypocrisy and yet full with blessings.

*When we were leaving, Clara said she would make another pie in the fall, when apples and pears were in season and that she'd love to come to my house and we could eat the pie there. She said she loved driving to the other side of the mountain and looking at all the large old homes on River Road. But time went by quickly that fall and winter came much earlier than anyone expected so that as early as mid-October it was snowing almost every day and since Clara is afraid to drive in bad weather she didn't come that fall or winter either and our friendship was sustained through telephone calls. She said she never made the pie either, that it was not the right object or subject to photograph in winter, and instead she photographed her boots and overcoat; vases on tables, empty of flowers; trees without leaves; and the cornfields without corn growing. I listened well to her descriptions of the pictures. On account of my blindness my hearing is better than most people's. I hear the wind even when it's not blowing. I hear songs when they're not sung, conversations not said out loud, poems of inconsequence—overlooked or ignored by those who see with their eyes only. My vision is more mental but no less real. People are suspicious of that—*How can a blind person see?—*but Clara has faith in my sight. She says that when she explains her pictures to me, she sees them through my mind, as I see them, and that no one else sees them as well as me.*

My girlfriend had gone back to Jamaica to be with her family since her mother had become ill. I was lonely and the house with many rooms and many windows was always drafty and cold. Clara's calls were always welcomed and within her detailed descriptions of her pictures of winter clothes, winter skies, winter light, or winter moods—pictures that I can and cannot see—my loneliness and the loneliness of a long winter in a mountainous region where there is nowhere to walk to for companionship or even a newspaper, pervade.

Now that spring is here and what I long for I have not lost sight of, Clara will come. We will cry over how much we have missed each other and that another year has passed. She will tell me what she is wearing: whether it is asymmetrical, bell-, pear- or box-shaped; its color and fabric, age and story; whether it's masculine or feminine etc. I will tell her about Carl, the cat who climbed in through the window one very cold winter's night, took over my bed, and gave birth to five kittens, so that I realized that Carl was the wrong name for the cat and after that called her Carlotta. I will explain that Carlotta gracefully slipped out the same window she had come in, and took the kittens with her. She had stayed in a warm house on a comfortable bed long enough to give birth and provide a home for her babies, and then when it was warmer outside and the kittens old enough, they vanished, not even leaving one kitten behind.

Frances

I don't sleep through the night the way I used to, nor do I stay up all night and sleep the greater part of the day, also like I used to. Instead, I sleep in small amounts throughout the day: a little here, a little there. When I can't sleep at night I watch TV because I'm too tired to read. On TV is mostly news, which is mostly bad, and when I try to talk with Theo about the violence and poverty in the world he always tries to steer the conversation to more cheerful subjects.

Sometimes in the daytime I clean a drawer, or a section of the closet, or vacuum part of a room. In that way, I clean much like I sleep, in pieces. I eat like this, too: half a banana in the early morning, the other half in the late morning; one cup of tea in the afternoon, another cup in the late afternoon; half a bowl of soup for dinner and the other half before the night is through. So rather than sleeping through the night, cleaning the entire apartment, or eating a whole meal, through small efforts I manage to eat and sleep enough while keeping my surroundings clean.

Theo wants me to come and live with him. He and his wife Clara live in a cabin in the woods in Pine Forest with their two cats and no TV. The ceiling of my apartment in New York City leaks whenever it rains and in winter there's often little or no heat. I have one mouse that lives in the kitchen that I rarely see but hear when I'm laying in bed at night.

The mouse is eating a bar of soap that I forgot to cover. My son advises me to get a cat. He says the smell of the cat would encourage the mouse to move elsewhere, but that would be another attachment to add in this time of life for letting go. Besides, what will happen to the cat when I die or move from the apartment? For these reasons, you'd think I'd want to live in Pine Forest; but I want to stay here. I don't want to make any changes nor do I want to have to adjust. I'm hard of hearing. I play the TV loud, and the first thing that Theo does when he comes to visit, even before taking his coat off, is to turn the volume down. He doesn't understand that I play it that loud in order to hear it. I would have to explain that to him and Clara if I were living with them. I'm not interested in explaining myself. I'm interested in what can't be explained.

Clara

When Clara returned from her travels in India, the first thing Theo told her was what he was reading. Funnily enough, he was reading a spiritual book and not a novel. The book was written by an American named Samuel Lewis, one generation older than Theo, yet Theo had met him once. Sam was a Sufi, a member of an order of dervishes that believed that the soul, which is unchanging and undying, is the observer, who stays in the back of the background watching. This watcher of change, and the changes are many, remains pure and is one's true nature. Through the experience of ecstatic dance, which Sam dedicated his life to, the watcher within the dervish emerges out of the background, and the dancer is unveiled.

Other themes, besides dance, in his book were invocations. Theo said that, according to Sam, an invocation usually starts with the mind turned toward a specific object such as Mary, Buddha, Allah, Krishna, Yahweh, etc., but that a specific object is not necessary because the Supreme Being that one calls to is ultimately beyond form and omniscient so that one can enter into an attitude or atmosphere of devotion without a concrete object or many objects, specific or not. Clara smiled as she listened to Theo's thoughts about his book, knowing that if she herself were to read it, it would not be as clear to her as hearing his interpretations. That night, in the low light of their small and unassuming cabin, Theo lit up Clara's mind in the way that the light of a candle reaches to the four corners of a room. This light brightened everything that was a part of it, making it easy to see the distinction between what is important and what is not.

Isaac and Martha

Soon after Clara returned from India, her neighbors Isaac and Martha came over to say *hello*. They hadn't traveled much and were curious to hear about India. As Clara described Sarana, she realized that her viewpoint was one-sided. Clara did not mention the fact that there are children who are abandoned, grow up in orphanages, and at puberty are sold for prostitution; nor did she mention that she actually knew someone who'd helped expose this corruption, who now had to live in hiding, since the one she exposed was released after only two months in jail. She did not mention that bulls are whipped to make them pull their wagons quickly, or that cows are borderline starving and only fed enough to provide milk for people.

Instead, she talked about how safe she felt in the middle of the night in a shantytown, where the bus stopped and everyone got off for a cup of tea. She talked about haggling with a vendor over the price of something and then immediately after the price was settled having a friendly conversation with him. She talked about the smell of jasmine and curry instead of that of human sewage and garbage floating down the river. She knew in the back of her mind as she heard herself telling her neighbors about India that something was missing with the picture she painted, that it was incomplete. Clara wondered how her neighbors pictured the images she was describing. She knew it couldn't be the same as what she'd seen because her viewpoint was singular and personal; but she also knew that consciousness is shared. To see everything all at once and simultaneously in its entirety and understand it is what Clara imagined it was to be enlightened.

Isaac and Martha told Clara that while she was in India they were busy making maple syrup, as it was March; and the hope was, at that time of year, to have warm days and cold nights. But March turned out to be quite cold in the daytime so the syrup wasn't flowing. Meanwhile, four of their

Book IV: The Rain Cloud

eight cats had an allergic reaction and their ears were swollen and they were sneezing. The doctor gave the cats cortisone shots and Martha cleaned the house; but what they were allergic to couldn't be determined and they continued sneezing. Besides that, their refrigerator had broken and Isaac had ordered a part in the hopes of saving some money and the refrigerator. But while they waited for the part to arrive, Martha had a feeling it might not be the right part. As Clara listened to the problems of her friends, India seemed far away. But at night in her sleep she dreamed of the shantytown and the cup of tea and was almost a little surprised to wake and find Theo and the two cats next to her and that she was no longer in Sarana.

Moses

While Clara was away, Moses made a movie based on the tragedy in his family when he was twelve. He sent out a mass letter asking if anyone had had a similar tragedy, where one had been affected by the suicide of a close one. Clara's mother Sarah had known of several cases in Germany when the Gestapo came and a member of the family asked if they could go to the bathroom, where they ingested cyanide and died that way instead of being carried off to the death camps. Clara wondered whether that would be considered suicide and if the mind was perhaps in a clear state when making that choice. Clara thought Moses's idea for the movie was a good one and that it would help him as well as the others who answered his email to create something positive from their suffering. This was the beauty of the mind when it is used properly; it becomes an instrument for healing.

Clara

Clara herself had known three people who'd taken their own lives, but not because the Gestapo was waiting at the front door. There, the reasons were more personal, emotional, and depressive, revolving around low self-worth and substance abuse. Clara was not close with them, but nonetheless had wondered afterwards whether she could have done something to change the outcome of these events, had her own mind been more acute. She did not even know at the time what was going on, and for that a feeling of responsibility lingered. Similarly but different, as she grew older and knew more people who had not killed themselves but who through other causes had left this world, Clara realized that she missed them more than when they were alive. Even those she had not known well or strangely enough disliked: just knowing they were no longer around, that she wouldn't bump into them ever again, affected her.

Was it love? Was love more present in all of her relationships than she realized? Was this true of everyone? Was this the condition of ignorance: not knowing one's capacity for love, not understanding its fluidness? After her travels, Clara was in the mood to ask herself such questions. She wondered if she was missing those who were no longer there because they were part of herself: here not here, anywhere or elsewhere. Was she a shifting changing reality, made up of all that was around her and not around her, within all of which was one substratum? And was that all along love?

Clara's consciousness turned toward the memories and impressions from her trip to India. Her friends in Mumbai had taken her to a luxurious restaurant in a modern and expensive part of the city. When the waiter asked if she would like anything to drink she asked for a glass of wine. The waiter answered that no alcohol was served at the restaurant and Clara was confused. It seemed to Clara that all restaurants with extensive menus and expensive prices in modern cities served alcohol. The waiter explained that this was actually a Buddhist restaurant connected to a monastery and that many of the workers, though not dressed in traditional robes, were actually monks dressed in semi-lay clothes, still brownish red in color, because it was easier to work in them. Clara was embarrassed and assured the waiter that there had been no real desire for a glass of wine, that it was just a fleeting thought, now completely gone, and that she was happy to be in a Buddhist restaurant.

The waiter seemed upset that he could not serve Clara what she'd requested. A few minutes passed and the waiter returned with a wine glass full of wine. He set it down on the table in front of Clara, smiled, and disappeared. Clara was surprised. She lifted the glass and took a sip. Inside the glass was grape juice. She drank the grape juice. All along, it might as well have been wine, for the way it made her feel a little drunk. Once in her system, it turned to alcohol, maybe brandy . . . dandelion, pear, or apple. Clara was thinking of the mind of the waiter and wanted a mind like his. Or was her mind already like his: for hadn't it been her viewpoint of the waiter and the grape juice that had caused her intoxication?

From that recollection came other past recollections, mixing new with old. She hung the new clothes her tailor had made in the closet with the old ones and went downstairs to eat lunch. She thought about how the whole of her life was made up of combinations: socks and shoes, broccoli and brown rice, soap and water, restaurants and friends.

She thought of other combinations—starvation and gluttony, poverty and excess, fear and safety, sickness and health, young and old, inhalation and exhalation, life and death—sometimes with only a fine line separating them. She looked away from her lunch at her cat Hazel and thought, *Who chose to put the tree with a leaf? A flower with a bee? A cloud with rain?* She looked out of the window at the white snow around her cabin as daylight began to turn toward evening. The treetops were swaying and the ground remained still.

She thought of other combinations: fresh air coming in through a window cracked open by a nurse in a stuffy hospital room; love moving through the passengers on an airplane during serious turbulence; soldiers on opposite sides, "enemies," who would kill each other on the battlefield, on a day off from war as at Christmas or New Year's, playing chess on the would-be "front line." For Clara, these juxtapositions were understood, celebrated, unified, and left in the novels and essays of Virginia Woolf, symbolized mostly in the character of Clarissa Dalloway, who carefully prepares the menu, hems the curtains, decorates the rooms, arranges the flowers, and sets the table for her party, amidst tragedy, war, uncertainty, mental illness, and the fear of possible explosions. These are the juxtapositions, mixtures, gradations, differences, and similarities of a spider making its web from the cavity in the center of the heart known as the soul, the conscience, providing the ability to purify oneself and find one's Self in the middle and midst of one's life.

Clara had the feeling that her insights, as obvious as they may have seemed, were pivotal. She thought about the infinite possibilities in the natural world. Sitting at the kitchen table, she saw all the moments and events that had made up her life, as if using a microscope and telescope, giving her the ability to see better, to enlarge, bring close, make clear, unobstruct, and illuminate. She looked to the right and left, in the mirror, out the window, and back through the sediment of her mind. She saw, like dance movements or musical pieces, groups of people; arrangements of elements; aggregates of sequences and circumstances; collections of fabrics, handkerchiefs, and old blue plates—until the colorings and moods flowing through her mind ceased. She drifted fast and slowly, all at once and gradually toward what had been there all along, inside and everywhere, the uncovered universe, Love Supreme. She rested there, present, without the past and future pulling her, in an exulted state. There was no absence of anything.

Afterwards, she picked up her sewing. She had a few items she'd wanted to repair for some time. She rejoiced in the connection between the cloth and her hands and with her eyes she followed the movement of the needle and its thread, up, over, under, and across. In a small old wooden chair, she was sitting, sewing and happy.

THE YOGA SUTRA OF PATANJALI

I.I   In the auspiciousness of the present moment, the experience of yoga is alongside of, behind, before, connected to, in the direction of, and near to these sacred and poetic instructions.

I.2   The mental field of consciousness is unbiased and unlimited. When consciousness stops identifying itself with the ups and downs in life, then there is yoga. Yoga is (known, experienced, recognized) when the thought waves (*vrittis*) that superimpose themselves on the mental field are understood, controlled, set aside, not identified with, and not left to grow (*nirodah*).

I.3   Then, in the clear mind state, the experiencer becomes a seer, one who, like a guardian angel, watches over others, perceiving what is hidden, mysterious, and natural, and dwells in a place for learning.

I.4   Otherwise, one is absorbed in and identifies with one's mental waves, and what lies underneath remains so covered that one is only aware of what is on the surface, and is preoccupied with illusions.

I.5   There are five ways in which the mind turns and whirls in waves; they are painful or not painful, disturbing or not disturbing, and can cause one to feel artificial, impaired, unhealthy, tired, afflicted, tormented, impotent . . . or not.

1.6 The whirlings and turnings of the mind are composed of right knowledge, wrong knowledge, imagination, sleep, and memory.

1.7 Right knowledge or forward thinking is made up of that which is seen directly with one's own eyes, that which is not seen directly but can be inferred through a sign or clue, and that which is communicated through a reliable source such as a teacher or scripture, so that what one can't see or even infer is acquired through a transmission.

1.8 Wrong or mistaken knowledge is to see the form or appearance of something erroneously, such that it appears different than what it really is.

1.9 Falling into a moment where one's mind is not limited to the confines of time is called imagination. Objects of sound, word, and language are empty and absent of any real object.

1.10 Thoughts, objects, and supports will continue to appear and disappear with the absence of ideas, assumptions, credibility, or proofs, in sleep even if they are not recollected upon awakening.

1.11 The capacity to store experiences and later recall them, such that thoughts that lie dormant resurface, is called memory.

1.12 To turn toward and sit with is practice (*abhyasa*). To turn away from, to separate or cut oneself off from, is nonattachment (*vairagya*). When we turn toward something, automatically, we turn away from something else. This is *abhyasa vairagya*, a practice for establishing *yogash chitta vritti nirodah*.

1.13 Practice (*abhyasa*) is made steady through determination, effort, perseverance, and great care.

I.14 What defines practice as a practice is that it takes place over a long period of time, without interruption, with earnestness and devotion. With these qualities, one's practice will establish and provide a solid ground or strong foundation to wisely build upon.

I.15 Full knowledge and mastery of what one wishes to master is the result of the state where the mind is not attached to, or thirsty for, worldly objects that one has seen or heard about. Life is no longer aimed at getting or having the things of the world. No longer addicted to desire, one does not linger after expectations, nor look to solve their problems through the material world.

I.16 At the higher level of *vairagya*, one no longer identifies with the qualities (*gunas*) of the world of change (*prakriti*), and instead identifies with the soul, that which underlies change, and therein the thirst for personal satisfaction in the manifest world is over.

I.17 A type of *Samadhi* that takes place as a result of *abhyasa vairagya* is called *samprajnatah*. *Samprajnata Samadhi* is an expansive harmonic knowledge that reveals one's true form (*rupa*) and is made up of levels, which form a chain, from gross to subtle. It is a process of turning inward, from effect to cause, and tracing a concrete object back to its true nature.

I.18 When the normal activity of the mind stops, what is left are the impressions of one's previous practice, going all the way back to ancient times. Practice leaves a residue (*samskara*) that sanctifies one's life beyond ordinary comprehension and creates a situation where the mind settles into a state of awareness, free of an object, support, or idea that one is aware of. Awareness, at this state, is called the "other" *Samadhi*, implying its indescribability.

I.19 This "other" *Samadhi*, at the further level, is without an awareness of one's body/mind entity, or one's temperament, disposition, and constitution. Here, at the subtlest level, the place of rest is no longer the finite form. Finally, the sense of limitation in one's name and form dissolves.

I.20 Other methods (other than *abyasa vairagya*) to bring about yoga (I.2) are: faith, stamina, memory, deep absorption, and insight.

I.21 The greater the intensity of practice the closer enlightenment will be.

I.22 One's practice is distinguished by measures of gentleness, moderation, and balance, and the ability to focus intensely.

I.23 There is a guiding principle (*Isvara*) that exists and works through names and forms, though a specific name and form is not given, e.g. Krishna, Jesus, Yahweh, God, etc. Thus, *Isvara* is not limited to name or form.

I.24 *Isvara* is untouched from the karmas (actions with consequences) done under the influence of misery, as the actions of *Isvara* are free of any selfish motive, even the slightest of all. *Isvara* is a special soul who can change circumstances for the better and manifests entirely for the benefit of others.

I.25 The seed to all knowledge exists within the relationship between the devotee and *Isvara*. The experience of dedicating one's actions to *Isvara* or feeling *Isvara*'s presence is a shelter, home, and safe place where one can take rest and no danger will come.

I.26 *Isvara* is the *guru* from before, the remover of darkness, the guiding principle, not limited to time. When the force of *Isvara* is strong within a particular form, the tradition is to call that form *guru*. *Isvara* may appear at any time, in any place, in any form, as a special soul, when darkness is overwhelming.

1.27 *Isvara* has a name and can be called upon. The sound of this name is described as *pranavah. Pranavah* refers to the syllable AUM, and means the sound of renewal, as it cuts through the chitter chatter in our minds, which keeps us from experiencing the present moment. The name is a way of voicing praise. Since AUM does not appear in the text itself, it is implied that there are other words and sounds that spiritual traditions use as a name and link to this guiding principle.

1.28 The meaning and purpose of AUM is searched for, remembered, created, and realized through the external and internal repetition of AUM. The meaning unfolds through the recitation.

1.29 From that (realization of the meaning of AUM *pranavah*) comes a special state of consciousness where one, in a deep state of meditation on the sounds of *Isvara*, relinquishes all distractions. In this restful state of awareness, one becomes learned and is conscious of a central unity amongst all sentient beings. This mastery stands in the way of obstacles that would prevent one's enlightenment. The obstacles have no way of penetrating through this special state of consciousness, and, in time, disappear completely.

1.30 The obstacles are: sickness, dullness, doubt, carelessness, laziness, lack of affection, wrong vision, inability to focus, ability to focus but without sustaining it. These nine obstacles are signs that one's mind is not turned toward, or absorbed in, *Isvara* (the force of spiritual guidance).

1.31 The symptoms that go along with the obstacles listed above are: pain, depression, shakiness, and difficulty breathing. A mind that gets depressed has a lot of negativity and gets irritated easily. These conditions show that the mind is scattered and fragmented.

1.32 The prevention of the above listed symptoms and distractions takes place by removing their causes and putting practices in their place.

These practices, though there may be many, have one underlying, essential, principle purpose: to remember one's true nature, the Self, and to remove the obstacles of that remembrance.

I.33 By friendliness for those who are happy, compassion for those who are suffering, joy for those who are virtuous, and neutrality for those without virtue, one's mind realizes graciousness, kindness, and serenity, and becomes like blessed food.

I.34 (Another way of removing the obstacles that prevent enlightenment) is by retaining one's breath out after the exhalation; expelling one's breath out and restraining, stretching, and holding in the life force. (Another way of removing the obstacles that prevent one's enlightenment) is through awareness of the life force, carried within our breath. The mental waves (*vrittis*) are suspended through the use of the breath. Exhale retention grants one a restored feeling of gratitude for life and breath as its sustainer, especially when one inhales afterward.

I.35 (Another way of causing the removal of the obstacles listed above [I.30–31] and suspending the negative *vrittis* ...) is holding the mind on a tangible object so that that activity of the mind causes a mental state of progress and refinement. Once the subtlety of the object is perceived, the subtlety of one's cognition is realized as well. Using the mind to focus on an object, to move from gross to subtle, from physical to essential, in an orderly way, is an expansive form of thinking, and a more authentic mental state than the conditioned or fragmented ways thoughts often fluctuate. The unobstructed perceiver of an object, in this case, becomes a seer and one with peace of mind.

I.36 (Serenity of mind comes from) a measure of bright light which separates you from sorrow.

I.37 By placing the mind on an object that is gentle and free of attachments, one attains a similar state of mind.

I.38 Knowledge that comes to us by way of dreams and deep sleep can be a support for enlightenment.

I.39 Concentrate and meditate on that which is most esteemed or longed for.

I.40 The mastery that comes from mental ease and brightness (*chitta prasadanam*) gives one the ability to extend oneself beyond measure in any way one wishes.

I.41 When the mental whirlings (*vrittis*) thin out, the mind approaches nobility and becomes clear, like a well-polished gemstone, and the seer, seen, and act of seeing coincide and honor each other. The seer comes to see him- or herself through what he or she sees. The knower comes to know him- or herself through knowing what he or she knows. The experiencer comes to experience him- or herself through experiencing what he or she experiences. This merger is known as *samapattih*, an unexplained experience of events falling perfectly into place.

I.42 Words, sounds, names, notes, and songs (*shabda*); meaning, significance, and purpose (*artha*); knowledge, what is known, learned, and understood (*jnana*); ideas, doubts, and imaginations (*vikalpa*), questions, analyses, reasoning, and inquiry (*savitarka*) form combinations, so that the experiencer has an inexplicable experience of unity, not willed upon.

I.43 Most of what is remembered, recalled, or recollected is biased and colors the way one sees what is in front of one. When these obscurations are removed, through the processes of purification, what is seen and its purpose shine, and the seer is free from thoughts. A direct experience is one where the experience is not experienced through the filter of one's memories. A direct experience is one where the experiencer feels as if they are not there. When one's memory is purified, one is as if empty of one's own appearance, character, condition, nature, aims, shape, and form.

(In the previous sutra a state of mind is described where merger occurs with thought through positive logic—*savitarka*. In this sutra a subtler state is described, one without thought, where thoughts are no longer purposeful—*nirvitarka*.)

I.44 More mystical, refined, and intangible realms are experienced with and without the fluctuations of the mind. The subtlety of perception of an object of affection keeps increasing with and without the movements of the mind. Subtle hidden qualities of objects are revealed within realms of concentration beyond ordinary thought.

I.45 Through the work of clearing the mind, that which differentiates one from another loses its dominance. Through the work of clearing the mind, one's perceptions extend from gross to subtle and still subtler levels of names and forms until finally one perceives the subtlest level, which is nameless, formless, and not different in any way from any other. At this underlying level, the world is subtle, simple, and unmarked.

I.46 These (*samapattih* states)—*savitarka* (with thought), *savichara* (with reflection), *nirvitarka* (without thought), *nivicara* (without reflection)— are seeds to enlightenment (*Samadhi*). The reality that lies beyond name and form is experienced as a result of a seed.

I.47 Beyond inquiry is the clear, unerring wisdom of the supreme Self, which is full of beauty. When one's concentration on an object extends to the subtlest level of the object, it will no longer be necessary to hold onto the object. When the object is released, and the mind is empty of supports, the impermanent nature of all that passes is accepted and one rests in the kindness and fullness of one's divine nature.

I.48 The wisdom and intuition there (beyond inquiry) is truth fulfilling (*rtambara*). From gross to subtle, with and without object, with and without supports, with and without inquiry, to a state beyond inquiry, unfolds the ability to perceive truth at the universal level. From one state to another, turning to a greater truth, by letting go of concepts, beliefs, words, memories, illusions, and bias.

I.49 The intuition that comes as a result of the experience of universal truth is distinct from what one has heard, read, inferred, or learned via traditions, as this final knowledge is innate. *Visesa*—insight that comes to us when the mind is at rest.

I.50 The impressions that turn into tendencies (*samskaras*) that come from the truth-bearing state (*rtambara*) prevent the acting out of other tendencies coming from previous impressions from sprouting. This is how we change. Finally, all one is left with is the seed of enlightenment.

I.51 Of that (the *samskara*) of the truth-bearing state (*rtambara*) is the seed (*bija*) that stops the growth of seeds. Without seed (*nirbija*), with nowhere else to go, the bright light of awareness (*chit*) not aware of an object other than itself, is self illumined. This is the seed of self-realization. The seed without a seed. Each level of perception plants the seed for the next level until finally all the past seeds are wiped out and no new seeds are planted. One is not burdened by the past or pulled into the future. One is free to absorb the other into oneself and experience *Samadhi*.

* * *

2.1   Hard work beyond one's ordinary capacity (*tapas*), the study of one's divine nature and the application of that study (*svadyaya*), and devotion to the *Guru*/God/Enlightenment principle are three actions that when combined become actions of purification.

2.2   The purpose of these purifications is to make thin, starve, emaciate, and not feed one's afflictions (*kleshas*) and thereby realize enlightenment (*Samadhi*).

2.3   One who is unaware of the Self (*avidya*), will identify oneself with a name and form other than the Self (*asmita*); will suffer from excessive craving (*raga*), excessive avoiding (*dvesha*), and an underlying fear of all that is changing, coming–going, and dying (*abhinivesha*).

2.4   The absence of self-knowledge (*avidya*) is a fertile field where other miseries grow. The extent to which this ignorance influences one's actions varies from present without expression, asleep but there in the germ form, to and/or mild, alternating, on and off, or fully rising and active. Misery is a projection that grows out of the field of not knowing the Self. When one recognizes the Self in others, one will recognize the Self in oneself.

2.5   Ignorance (*avidya*) causes us to mistake the impermanent for the permanent, the impure for the pure, and pain for joy.

2.6   When the power of the seer and the power of seeing seem as if made up of one, this is egotism. The seer identifies with the ability to see because of the ego.

2.7   Alongside of happiness is the craving for more happiness.

2.8   Alongside of pain is the hatred of pain.

2.9 One's own inclination toward life and away from death flows and grows strong, even in the wise. The predicament of the ultimate pairing of life and death, which stems from *avidya*, is a source of great worry and distress, even for the wise. Without a sense of one's Self, beyond the mind/body entity, one will not be prepared for death.

2.10 The five afflictions are resolved back to their source through a backward motion. The direction that one is moving in can be reversed at any time.

2.11 The *kleshas*, in their subtlest form, exist as thoughts that are to be abandoned, or ended, through meditation (*dhyana*).

2.12 The foundation of our suffering is stored in the form of karma, where it will be experienced in the births, seen and unseen. In the lifetime that is seen and in future lifetimes, the storehouse, mansion, stomach, and/or bedroom of karma has its root in the five afflictions and is experienced in present (seen) and future (unseen) births.

2.13 Actions undertaken when influenced by ignorance are the result of previous actions undertaken under the influence of ignorance. As long as those actions and their afflictions exist, their consequences or fruits will develop, ripen, and manifest through species, circumstances, and life span in future births. Past actions plant seeds that accumulate and are saved in the storehouse of karmic seeds, where they eventually, when the circumstances are right, ripen. This ripening distinguishes future birth, its length and quality, and the type of experiences one has. Worldly existence and its three-fold conditions—birth, length, and quality—are determined by karma.

2.14 These births will result in joy, delight, and auspiciousness, or sorrow, agony, and inauspiciousness, according to the virtuous or non-virtuous nature of their causes.

2.15 The three sources of pain are change, anxiety, and habit. One's mind is conflicted when the qualities of one's thoughts are not in harmony with one's nature. For the discerner (the one who can separate the Self from the nonself, the invisible spirit from the visible world), everything that changes is painful. Mistaking one's Self for the changing rather than the changeless is powerful, and out of it comes misery in all directions.

2.16 Suffering that has not yet come is avoidable. Future suffering is to be avoided. In order for future suffering to be avoided, perpetrating cycles that cause suffering must stop. Suffering that has not yet come can be avoided by not creating it. By understanding the relationship between cause and effect (*karma*), future suffering can be ended.

2.17 The cause of future suffering is the mistaken identification of the seer with the seen. The cause of future suffering is the union of the seer with the changes the seer sees. What the seer sees is caused by the karmas of the seer.

2.18 The seen exists for the purpose of providing experience and spiritual fulfillment. Learning from what we live through leads to a final fulfillment. The perception or reading of an experience is influenced by one's state of mind made up of serenity, activity, and dullness. A complete experience is one where the habitual way of seeing is abandoned, so that the fulfillment of the experience becomes a release from conditioned or rigid ways of seeing. The seen is made up of elements perceived through the senses. The elements include water, air, fire, earth, and space, as well as all beings and creatures, including ghosts and spirits. The seen is shaped and influenced by the tendencies and dispositions of the mind of the seer, be it serenity, activity, or dullness. There is a relationship between the elements and the sense organs.

2.19 The seen world (*prakriti*) is perceived in four stages from manifest to un-manifest. The four stages are: 1. distinct, visible, accepted; 2. not distinct, invisible, subtle, universal; 3. only leaving a visible mark; 4. without a mark, undefined, formless vibration. Consciousness moves through these four stages. The stages of consciousness experienced determine how and what the seer sees.

2.20 The seer witnesses what the seer sees and thinks, while all along remaining pure. The purity and genuineness of the seer stays the same. The seer is not subject to the changing phenomenon.

2.21 The seeable exists only for the purpose of the seer.

2.22 Once the seer sees oneself in the seen, the purpose of the seen is accomplished, but the seen does not cease because it still has a purpose for others. Once the seer has accomplished seeing oneself in the seen, the seen does not cease to exist, nor is it wasted or lost.

2.23 Through the relationship between the seen and changing world and the seer, both are fully realized. Through contact with another, one finds the other in oneself.

2.24 The sense of otherness is perceived because of ignorance, later one realizes there is no other.

2.25 The disappearance of ignorance causes the disappearance of the union between the changeless seer and the changing phenomenon. The changeless seer, detached from identifying with all that is seen, stands alone and free. When one sees oneself in others, there will no longer be others to unite with. When one is no longer under the influence of ignorance (avidya), oneness replaces duality. This is called kaivalyam.

2.26 The flowing and continuous identification with the unseen One-ness is the means to completely end the confusion between the world of name and form and the invisible substratum, or Divine, underneath.

2.27 The dissolution of ignorance comes in seven levels. The wisdom of the seer unfolds in seven stages. The dawning of the illumination of Self happens in seven steps.

2.28 The impurities of one who undertakes, establishes oneself, and remains engaged in the limbs of yoga will diminish, and the light of knowing the real from the unreal will be kindled and beautified.

2.29 These are the eight limbs: *yama, niyama, asana, pranayama, pratyahara, dharana, dhyana, samadhi.* (This is the Royal Road. The first four limbs are sometimes described as the seeds for the last four.)

2.30 The five components of *Yama* are: *ahimsa, satya, asteya, brahmacharya, aparigraha. Yama* means twin, signifying the concept of two. The *yamas* are necessary for one who lives in a world of duality and wants to get enlightened, offering a support system for living while causing the least harm possible in every circumstance. *Ahimsa* is nonviolence. It includes not killing, but includes all lesser forms of violence as well. *Satya* is truthfulness usually associated with speech. *Asteya* is not stealing or taking things for granted. *Brahmacharya* is honoring the Creative Force and not abusing others sexually. *Aparigraha* is not grabbing for things excessively, not taking more than one needs, and thereby leaving enough for others. It's the path of non-accumulation. It is not taking now for later.

2.31 The practice of *yama*, made up of the five components, is The Great Vow as it relates to the whole world. It is to be practiced irrespective of birth, place, time, and or circumstance.

2.32 *Niyama* is that which supports *Yama* and is also made up of five components, which are *saucha, santosha, tapas, svadhyaya, Isvara Pranidhana.* *Saucha* is cleanliness in regards to one's inner and outer world. *Santosha* is contentment or acceptance of what is. Metaphorically, it is the worship of a small grain. *Svadhyaya* is one's own study of the Self and its application. *Isvara Pranidhana* is devotion to a higher, supreme force of guidance.

2.33 When disturbing thoughts arise, meditate and realize their opposite. Suspend the thoughts that are damaging to yoga and counter them through contemplating the other side. Rather than dwelling in negative thought waves, raise an opposing wave.

2.34 Negative thoughts that cause violence that one directly participates in, or does not directly participate in but accepts and/or approves of, may be mild, moderate, or intense, and will result in the fruits of endless misery and lack of spiritual knowledge. Thus, rest in the thoughts that are contrary to the disturbing thoughts.

2.35 In the presence of one who is completely established in nonviolence, all violence ceases. The one who continuously practices nonviolence creates an atmosphere of nonviolence and awakens love in the hearts of those in his or her presence. Thus, the result of one's practice is seen in one's world.

2.36 When the aspirant becomes established in truthfulness he or she develops an insight into how karma works and thus understands what the fruits of his or her actions will be. Thus, what he or she says will come true and will benefit the destiny of the world.

2.37 When one is established in non-stealing and renders one's entire mind in unconditional universal honesty, one obtains all prosperity.

2.38 When one moves in harmony with the creative spirit, one attains great courage and vitality. When one uses their creative powers to expand the things of beauty, an electrical force works through them.

2.39 Everything that one has that one doesn't need takes up unnecessary space in the subconscious of one's minds. When one unburdens the subconscious, the contents of the mind unfold. Upon a foundation of non-hoarding, one understands the reason for one's birth. If one gives up traveling with more than one can carry and goes with what one can manage, one will know the purpose of traveling.

2.40 When one's own bodily parts are pure, the impure bodily parts of others are non-threatening. One is not touched or fearful of darkness when one is light. An enlightened one is not at risk of becoming contaminated.

2.41 On purity of *sattva*, one is continuously inspired, has established single-pointed focus, and has mastery over their senses. Thus, one is prepared for self-realization.

2.42 There is no greater gain or achievement than to worship the smallest particle of creation as the greatest source of happiness. The capacity to be thankful is linked to *citta vrtti nirodah*; that which is inside makes that which is outside enjoyable to us. Knowing this, one is content. On account of this high level of contentment, a transcendental bliss is easily found, arises naturally, and leaves one desire-less.

2.43 When one is entirely focused on one's spiritual practice (*sadhana*), the gross impurities diminish and the bodily sense organs are made perfect. When one welcomes challenges as blessings, one's super powers are heightened. In the same way that laziness diminishes our capabilities, hard work increases our capabilities. Knowing this one is not afraid to work hard. One who practices austerities can see, hear, taste, touch, and smell what is normally out of the reach of the sense organs.

2.44 The study, worship, and contemplation of one's own chosen deity causes the union of oneself to that deity, who then comes to them in their dreams, thoughts, and in other ways as well.

2.45 By offering oneself to one's chosen personal highest supreme divine form of guidance, one achieves and perfects *Samadhi*. Thus, *Samadhi* is attained through devotion.

2.46 One's seat or connection to place, space, earth, and or support is described as firm, unmoving, elastic, unfettered, settled, balanced, steady, consistent, natural, poised, composed, solid, secure, stable, certain, not rigid, and to provide or make happy, joyful, comfortable, centered, at ease, and established in a good space and location. *Asana* is a seat that is close to the earth and is a position of worship, humility, concentration, meditation, and love.

2.47 Effort, effortlessness, and a feeling of infinity bring a level of *samadhi* through *asana*. Effort turns to effortlessness, force turns to without force, and the awareness of oneself at the deeper level is experienced where one is no longer separate from the cosmic flow of the life force.

2.48 Thus, one is no longer afflicted by pairs of opposites and released from, "I like this; I don't like that."

2.49 Thus, the motion of one's inhalation and exhalation is controlled, expanded, regulated, suspended. . . . While the mastery of *asana* is there, one can stop the flow of inhale and exhale and control the movement of the breath.

2.50 The breath may be stopped externally, internally, or midway, and regulated according to place; climate, diet, time; time of day, time of year, time in relation to lengths of breaths.

2.51 The fourth condition is beyond the three conditions—place, time, number; inhale, exhale, in-between—where the outside air inside and the inside air outside no longer exist as essentially different.

2.52 As a result of the *pranayama*, the shroud over the internal light is removed and destroyed so that one is shining.

2.53 On account of this purity and non-hindrance of one's natural light, the mind will be capable for the next steps. Step by step this readiness is acquired.

2.54 When the mind is not fragmented, the sense organs become the mind's servant and thereby reflect the mind's true nature.

2.55 As a result of that, one gains supreme control over one's sense organs.

* * *

3.1 Concentration (*dharana*), holding the mind in a collected way, comes by way of directing, connecting, tying, locking, and keeping the mind energetically to or on a point, place, object, or seed that one feels affection or reverence for.

3.2 Meditation is when the concentrated mind continuously flows in one unbroken stream, without interruptions, toward a single idea or point of attention, solid or not.

3.3 *Samadhi* (absorption) is when meaning, significance, and purpose alone shine, illuminate, and make clear, as if empty of one's own form.

3.4 *Samyamah* is when the group of three (*dharana, dhyana, samadhi*) turn into one simultaneously or one to the other.

3.5 Due to the glory of *samyamah*, one sees, with insight, the world.

3.6 The application of the yoga of *samyamah* occurs in stages unfolding and involving new and distinct levels.

3.7 The group of three are the inner limbs distinct from the five limbs that came before.

3.8 Even that (the group of three) is an external limb of *Samadhi* without a seed.

3.9 When one's existing consciousness is maintained and stabilized in the space between mental impressions, where one mental impression has finished and a new one has not yet begun, and the movement of the mind is suspended, the consciousness experiences an all-pervasive transformation called *nirodah parinamah*.

3.10 From that (*nirodah parinamah*), the repeated impression that is peaceful, composed, quiet, and restful flows.

3.11 As distractions diminish and single-pointed focus takes its place, the mind transforms. This is called *samadhi parinamah*.

3.12 When the seed of that breaks open the objects of distraction and the objects of focus merge, this is called *ekagrata parinamah*. The same peaceful impression keeps arising into the field of consciousness over and over.

3.13 From that (the understanding of the essential principle of transformation), the character, conditions, qualities, make up, and potential of any object that undergoes change (any sentient being; plant, animal, creature, human, god, including the elements—earth, fire, metal, water, air, ether—and the power of the sense organs) is explained.

3.14 The original substance of any object at any stage of change remains a constant throughout, be it undefined, unpredictable, manifested, unmanifested, disappeared, quiet, or at rest.

3.15 The cause for variety in change is that the sequence of events from one moment to the next varies and differs from one another.

3.16 *Samyamah* (*dharana, dhyana, Samadhi* combined) on the three transformations (*nirodah, Samadhi, ekagrata*) brings knowledge of the past and future. Through observing change, one sees how something was, what it is, and what it will be. Hence the fluidity of time.

3.17 Different sounds make up different sets of words with different meanings, interpretations, associations, and ideas superimposed on top of each other, causing confusion that is lifted by *samyamah* on the distinction of word meaning and idea such that one knows, hears, and comprehends the cries and sounds of all the creatures of the universe.

3.18 Through observing one's tendencies, one gains knowledge of one's actions from a previous birth.

3.19 One knows the thoughts of another.

3.20 One knows what is behind or beyond the concrete thoughts of another's mind.

3.21 By *samyamah* on the body's form one is able to grasp, suspend, and disconnect oneself from the light that reaches to the eyes of others, thereby making one's Self invisible. One can suspend their visibility by minimizing in density and maximizing in transparency.

3.22 By the above, sound and others can be made unperceptible, imperceivable, etc.

3.23 By *samyamah* on the speed in which karma ripens, the sequence of events being slow or fast, one can read the signs, indicators, and hints of what will be at the other end, the outcome (short term, long term, in this life, in another life, personal, impersonal, universal, heavenly).

3.24 Friendship is the source and origin of strength.

3.25 Through *samyamah* on the strength of an elephant, one attains the strength of an elephant.

3.26 By directing the light of one's refined thoughts toward the subtle, hidden, or distant, the subtle, hidden, or distant is revealed.

3.27 By *samyamah* on the sun, the supreme light, the Solar Deity, the *sushumna nadi*, one attains knowledge of the whole world, the universe, all planets, and planetary systems.

3.28 By *samyamah* on the moon, one attains the supreme wisdom: the full, confidential, complete, experiential knowledge of the arrangements, forms, appearances, logic, and placement of the clusters of stars.

3.29 By *samyamah* on the Pole Star—the star that is in a fixed place, non-moving, unchangeable, stable, constant, permanent, firm, and eternal—comes the knowledge of the movements and passageways of the stars.

3.30 By *samyamah* on the psychic navel center, one attains an understanding of the organization of one's body.

3.31 By *samyamah* on the well of the throat, hunger and thirst stop.

3.32 By *samyamah* on the subtle nerve channel named after the tortoise, one attains steadiness and balance.

3.33 By *samyamah* on the bright light of the crown on the head, one sees and has visions of those who have attained perfection.

3.34 Direct perception, without the use of the sense organs, illuminates everything.

3.35 By *samyamah* on the heart, one has complete knowledge of the mental field, the field of awareness, consciousness, intellect, feeling, and perception.

3.36 By *samyamah* on one's own purpose, distinct from the purpose of another, or one's highest purpose, distinct from other purposes, through the quality of brightness, *sattva*, the Self stands apart.

3.37 From that, hearing, touching, seeing, tasting, smelling without the use of the sensory organs (super sensory) arises.

3.38 The way of harming or abandoning one's *samadhi* is to use the accomplishments/powers (*siddhis*) while in an externalized state.

3.39 Through letting go of the causes of bondage, relaxing *karmic* ties, and remaining fluid in sensitivity and consciousness, one is able to leave one body and enter into and occupy the body of another.

3.40 Through mastery on the upward-moving, organic, *pranic*, energetic wind, one disassociates with water (rivers, streams, swamps, and ponds), earth (mud, clay, thorns, and the prickly parts of plants), and hovers, rises, ascends, is drawn up out of, and elevated in the most superior way in what is called levitation.

3.41 Through mastery of *samana* (the vital *pranic* energy concentrated and stored in the area of the navel psychic center that extends itself and moves to all body parts aiding in all kinds of digestion), radiance and illumination is kindled like a blaze or torch of intelligent, bright, glowing fire.

3.42 By *samyamah* on the relationship between hearing and the ethereal fluid pervading the whole universe, the sub-stratum of vibration, the sky, space, and atmosphere, one hears the divine celestial sounds of, within, and through the air.

3.43 By *samyamah* on the relationship between the body and the space the body exists in, one is able to make oneself light as cotton and travel through space.

3.44 When one stops imagining one's consciousness to be limited to one's name and form, there is a vivid light that releases, makes visible, uncovers, and diminishes what conceals, veils, and shuts out one's greater consciousness.

3.45 By *samyamah* on the natural order of states and objects, from the gross form to the essential, subtle, most hidden form, to the original form and divine purpose, one obtains mastery of all the elements, principles, and sub-strata.

3.46 From that, the power to reduce one's size to nothing, etc. (pass through fire like passing through air, walk on water like walking on earth, swim through earth like swimming through water), to manifest the body as perfect and be unafflicted and unobscured by the natural universal laws, results.

3.47 The body as perfect is described as beautiful, graceful, and strong like a diamond.

3.48 By *samyamah* on the relationship between the processes and action of perception, one's essential nature, one's sense of "I am," and the primary function and divine purpose of what one is grasping and why, comes mastery over the organs of perception.

3.49 From that, the speed of the mind transcends its instruments and without the need for a vehicle has mastery over the most important and excellent principle: inherent, predominant, the source of the material world, the primary germ out of which all material appearances evolve.

3.50 Through the awareness of the distinction between the *sattva*, purest, brightest, and closest state to the soul, *purusha*, and the *purusha* itself, one is the Supreme Knower of all things.

3.51 Through non-attachment (*vairagya*), even to this supreme state, comes the further diminishment of the seeds of obstructions of *kaivalyam*.

3.52 When approached with invitations from those in high places one must renew again and again one's lack of desire and pride for such contacts.

3.53 By *samyamah* on a single moment and the sequence of single moments the knowledge of discernment is born.

3.54 From that comes the knowledge of the differences of what appears similar in relation to an object's potential, beginning, and place.

3.55 This discerning knowledge where one instantly grasps all objects at the same time, beyond their sequential existence, beyond a place other than everywhere, causes the crossing of the ocean of conditional existence.

3.56 Thus, the purity of brightness and of the soul are equal, the same, and become each other, and this is enlightenment, *kaivalyam*.

* * *

4.1   Birth, herbs, mantra, austerities, and absorption bring forth the empowerments.

4.2   The transformations and changes that occur from one birth to the next are due to the overflowing nature of *prakriti*, the changing reality existing in the realm of name and form, made up of elements in combinations of qualities experienced by the sense organs.

4.3   The changing phenomena (the world, *prakriti*) is not the cause of enlightenment (*samadhi*) but is instrumental because of the inherent possibilities within change for uncovering veils and separating the unreal from the real, the passing from that which is eternal, like a farmer who does not cause the seed to sprout, as that is the seed's potential, but is through his work instrumental.

4.4   The identification with the finite individualized sense of "self" exists within that which is infinite and without measure.

4.5   Consciousness is one, but it divides into, directs, makes use of, and benefits many.

4.6   Of these (divided minds) the mind born of meditation is free from the storehouse of karmic seeds.

4.7   The karma of a *yogin*, unlike the karma of others, is neither white nor black, nor threefold.

4.8   From that, only the tendencies given the corresponding conditions will ripen and come to fruition.

4.9   Even the *samskaras*, karmic tendencies or impressions, seemingly separated by birth, place, and time, are without interruption, part of a continuous cycle that does not stop and start, and stored all as one in the depth of one's memory. Desires, thoughts, actions, and impressions from previous lives with different circumstances, stored in our memory, are influencing our present life as if there was no separation at all. A continuous memory recalls and integrates the previous lives, and events separate from the life one is previously having because of the oneness of memory.

4.10 Of these (*samskaras*) there is no beginning, end, or nonexistence as the expression of the wish for the blessing of life is continual, essential, and everlasting.

4.11 When the causes, supports, and shelters of the *samskaras* disappear, the *samskaras* will disappear.

4.12 Past and future exist in their own way, with their own characteristics and as different from each other. The past is over, the future has not yet come. Each exists owing to different possibilities of sequences of events.

4.13 They (the past and future) manifest, come into being, display themselves, become visible and distinct, and/or subtle, elusive, atomic, and minute, and belong to and are composed of the qualities of all substances in nature; hence, the suppleness of time.

4.14 The reality of an object is due to its unique path of change.

4.15 Due to the path of perception, the mind separates itself from the object it is perceiving and the two appear to be divided, breaking into two and existing in different and dualistic ways. The same object perceived by different minds will appear as different. Different paths will result in different views, along the way, even if at the end the object is the same.

4.16 What would happen to an object if the object is unobserved, unperceived, unwitnessed, and unrecognized?

4.17 An object is known or unknown by the way it colors one's mind. The colors of the objects one perceives mirror one's mind. The way one views an object is the way one views oneself. When an object colors one's mind, and the mind takes in the colors, the object becomes known or unknown depending on the degree of coloring.

4.18 The Self always perceives the activities of the mind without ever changing. The source, origin, soul, as it records, through consciousness, the plays upon it, remains in a state of changelessness.

4.19 That, the whirlings of the mind, is not self-illumined or self-reflective due to its seeable, observable nature.

4.20 And because of its (the thought waves) non self-illuminative nature, it cannot know itself. The Seer sees the object but the object cannot see itself.

4.21 One consciousness seen by another consciousness, one knower seen by another knower, is too many consciousnesses and too many knowers, causing one's memory to become confused. (Thus, though the thought waves and moods are many, consciousness is one.)

4.22 Consciousness assumes the form of its own intelligence through awareness of its unchanging nature. Something is known when one's own faculty of knowledge appears in a form that is without a sequence of events and unchanging in one's mental field.

4.23 All meanings, purposes, ideas, and objects in the mental field of consciousness are illumined by the Seer and colored by the seen.

4.24 The desires, attachments, impressions (*vasanas*) are unnumbered and varied and do not exist for their own sake but for the sake of and in collaboration with another.

4.25 The one who sees the Self as distinct carries the feeling of inactivity.

4.26 Then, that one whose mind is flowing with and downward from *viveka* moves without needing to be pushed, and without the weight of questions, desires, thoughts, karmas, etc. bends toward illumination.

4.27 When the easy flow of spiritual knowledge (*viveka*) breaks and splits open, other negative thoughts will still continue to arise due to the depth of past impressions, habits, tendencies, patterns, etc.

4.28 The way to remove those interfering thoughts will be the same as removing the kleshas as described earlier.

4.29 In a rapturous condition, without the weight of karma, one becomes light as a cloud of virtue, floating to the top, without ever again dropping down. The mind flows gracefully, without any force or effort, to enlightenment. The desire to gain anything of this world, or any other, evaporates into a state where there is no question of any desire, desires have no relevance, desires are extinguished into absolute happiness, and the removal of suffering turns to songs of praise, all naturally happening, like a rock falling down a hill or a tree branch leaning toward the ground on account of the heaviness of ripe fruit.

4.30 From this (*dharma megha Samadhi*), the actions motivated by afflictions and impurities tied to selfishness come to completion and end.

4.31 Then, with all the colorings, coverings, and imperfections removed, one's knowledge is infinite, all pervading, and what is left to learn is "little," almost nothing, negligible.

4.32 Because of that, the gunas and their processes of change, having fulfilled their purpose, come to closure in a final end.

4.33 At the other end, the uninterrupted sequence of events, made up of distinct moments, is easy to understand. Time will no longer be known as a devouring force but as providing a pathway that leads to perfection.

4.34 By the power of awareness of one's original form, the flow of change, empty of purpose, relaxes and recedes back to its source, leaving the soul, the *purusha*, untangled by changing phenomenon.

ACKNOWLEDGMENTS

My name is Ruth Gertrude Sidonia Lauer Manenti. Manenti is my husband's last name. Lauer is my surname. Sidonia and Gertrude were aunts of my fathers. Ruth is a Biblical name that both my parents liked. I am the wife of Robert Daniel Manenti and the daughter of Stefanie and James Lauer. My father's real name was Lothar, but when he escaped to this country as a refugee from Europe he changed his name to Jim. My father was a scientist and ran various highly respected laboratories. He worked in the field of physics, magnetics, and lubrication. He was the recipient of many grants and patents. He had students from all over the world. He suffered from terrible back and chest pain, worked hard his whole life, and passed on to me a strong work ethic. Though he had witnessed a great deal of violence having lived through World War Two, he was the kindest man I've ever known. My father passed away in 2009.

My mother is still alive. She is a writer. She has come to live near but not with me in a retirement community, and has made many new friends since her move. On Monday nights, she eats dinner with a group of men and women in their eighties and nineties and they only speak in French. Though my mother hadn't spoken French in decades, because of this one-night-a-week practice much of it has come back to her. On Thursday afternoons, she is in a play-reading group. They are currently reading *The Seagull* by Anton Chekhov: not one of her favorite plays by Chekhov, but nonetheless by Chekhov. My mother is exceedingly kind and generous. She has a great sense of humor and gets me laughing like no one else does. I treasure her company and influence. She remembers well most of Shakespeare's plays and poetry and can still recite long passages by heart. She is a great storyteller and if I have any gift at all for writing it directly comes from her. My brother Michael and his lovely wife Robin are both doctors, leaders in their fields, well liked and respected, humble, kind, good-natured, religious, and spiritual. My brother is also a vegan. They have two grown sons, one who studies rocket science and the other environmental biology.

My husband Robert has worked as a nurse for the last twenty-two years. He currently works in a small hospital in upstate New York where his patients appreciate him for his compassion, kindness, and genuine concern. He works with people who are very sick and often fragile. He likes people without wanting anything from them. He is gentle but firm. He likes the people he works with and they compliment him on his abilities to work well with others. He is a long-time, dedicated, and serious practitioner of Tai Chi. I have watched him practice diligently over twenty-one years of marriage. We have a wonderful marriage; it is a joy to live with him; he is an exceptional human being. We have two cats, Puffin and Mable. Puffin is the older: she is good-tempered and eats slowly. Mable is wilder and sometimes hisses at Puffin. They are loving and affectionate companions. My husband and I would find our cabin in the woods lonely without them.

None of this is really what I'm meant to be writing. I wanted to explain the nature of this book and how it relates to the *Yoga Sutra*. I wanted to thank the people who have in some way supported my work, and more precisely this book, but they are many in number. But keeping within the Indian tradition, a discourse on any subject usually includes a passage about the presenter of the subject, and that always starts by honoring one's family and teachers; for without them, the presenter would not exist.

I've been a student of yoga, both practice and theory, since 1985. My interest was stirred while I was recovering from a bad car accident, in which I broke many bones. My first lessons were from the boyfriend of one of the nurses who'd taken care of me when I was in the hospital. Later, after I moved to New York City, I attended classes at the Sivananda Yoga Vedanta Center on Twenty-fourth Street in Manhattan. In 1988, I enrolled in the Sivananda teacher's training course in India, which was primarily taught by Swami Shankarananda, who now goes by the name Robert Moses. One year later, when I was back in New York, I was introduced to Sharon Gannon and David Life, and since that introduction I have been their devoted student. It is hard to appropriately thank them or even in my own mind comprehend the blessings that have come to me through my association with them. They have set an example of the kindness, wisdom, and forbearance that comes from following with discipline, devotion, and integrity the practices of yoga. Without this example, my life and the lives of so many others would be totally different. They are the creators of the Jivamukti Yoga method, a path to enlightenment through compassion for all beings. I happily follow and teach this method, for which I am with each day increasingly more grateful.

In 1990, Sharon-ji, affectionately known as Padma, suggested I go back to India to meet Sri K. Pattabhi Jois, whom she said was a master of yoga. Shortly after our conversation, I took her suggestion, and in 1991 became a student and devotee of Guruji and of his daughter Saraswati and her son Sharath. Guruji left his body in 2009, so I had eighteen years of study with him in his physical form. That relationship was one of total trust. There are no words to express my gratitude for his consistent love and guidance. He was free of any pretense or ill will. As he acquired fame and wealth he remained the same simple, humble, sweet man.

In 1994, I heard Dr. M. A. Jayashree sing at a birthday party for Guruji. Her singing deeply affected me. When she was finished, I thanked her. She told me I would be able to sing too, and my first class with her was arranged for the next day at four PM. When I arrived, she was sleeping and I remember wanting the lesson so much that I woke her up out of a deep sleep. Since then, I have been a student of hers and her brother Narasimhan. They have taught me in particular the *Yoga Sutra*—how to chant it, and its meaning.

I am also a student of Professor H. V. Nagaraja Rao who also lives in Mysore, India (my home away from home)—the town where Guruji and Jayashree live. Professor Rao first started studying Sanskrit because he was too poor to go to the university, and at that time (the 1970s) the university was free to those who studied Sanskrit. There was also the added benefit of a daily meal ticket given to students studying Sanskrit. Of course, Professor Rao soon realized that the benefits were far greater than the initial motivations and later he became one of the most respected professors of Sanskrit in India and various other places in the world. That such a man would find time for me, welcome me into his home, and answer my simple questions is astounding to me. I have learned a great deal from him. I think it is important for students who meet their teachers when the teacher has already had some success to have an understanding of the difficulties and hard work that came before.

Andrea Boyd Cohen, who has enabled the projects I have undertaken to come to fruition, is my dear friend and editor of my two previous books. She agreed to help me with this third book and continued to help me even after I changed my mind, scrapped three years of our hard work, and started all over again. Her belief in the work and her desire to be of service was and is beyond what most people can fathom. She spent hours with me collaborating, looking for the right words, and making sure we weren't writing something offensive or incorrect in relation to the holy text. We pulled out all the dictionaries and other supporting books we could find, while her husband Jeffrey Cohen made us the most delicious popcorn in the world from his own secret recipe. Andrea is a gifted and compassionate yoga teacher and codirector with her husband of the Satsang Yoga school in Charleston, South Carolina. Working side by side on this project, over years, she has, for me, taken the word *friendship* to a new level and I treasure her and Jeffrey's presence in my life.

My best friend Lisa Schrempp went to Haiti after the terrible earthquake of 2010 and gave massages to two hundred children a day, for the three weeks that she was there. Because the situation in Haiti was declared a major disaster, she needed a doctor's note stating that she was in good health, in order to be granted permission to enter the country. Because of her thinness the doctor questioned her health. So she stood upside down on her hands and walked across the room and back, inspiring everyone around her with her strength. My friend Lois Conner is one of the greatest artists of all time. Her vision, skill, artistry, dedication, level of accomplishment, and humility need to be mentioned as they are highlights in my life and the lives of many. She has given me the key to her apartment and told me to think of her home as my own. Joel and Carol turn Stonybrook Road into a neighborhood where animals and trees are loved and cared for. Mark and Caren, whom we share the wild geese and the blue heron with, live close enough that someone kind and loving is always near. Rima Rabbath inspired the character of Gazelle. Her presence in my life is similar to that of Gazelle's in Clara's.

I wish to thank Jordon Pavlon, who read the manuscript carefully and gave great guidance and encouragement; Jessica Kung, for her ongoing help with my understanding of Devanagari and its transliterations; and Sharon Gannon who, in her usual way of suddenly having a great idea, came up with the title. It feels fitting that the title comes from Sharon, as a book without a title is like a person without a name. The depth of her support gives meaning to the name *Ruth*.

I wish wholeheartedly to thank Jeanine Munyeshuli Barbe, whose emails kept me going during an incredibly difficult time.

Special and most sincere gratitude to Martin Rowe, who was the first to speak of Clara, Theo, and Frances as real people whom he was genuinely interested in, who introduced me to the word *pericope* so I could have a better perspective of what I was doing; for publishing this book and two others; and through his brilliant edits, suggestions, and attention to detail making the books considerably better. Thank you Martin! Your support and patience are exceptional.

Further acknowledgments: Tomo Okabe, Susan Steiner, Jenn Morse, Geshe Michael Roach, Carlos Menjivar, the Gurudath family, Dr. Michael Lauer, Dr. Robin Avery, Jess Perry, Val Schaff, Krishna Kumari, Seane Corn, Yogeshwari, Susan Minot, John Brady, Barbara Pfister, Monica Jaggi,

Kelly Britton, Kimberly Flynn, Jules Febre, Ma Bhaskarananda, Ananda Ashram, and classical pianist Stephanie Brown—whose teacher's teacher's teacher's teacher's teacher's teacher's teacher was Beethoven.

I bow to the lotus feet of my guru, Sri K. Pattabhi Jois.

ABOUT THE AUTHOR

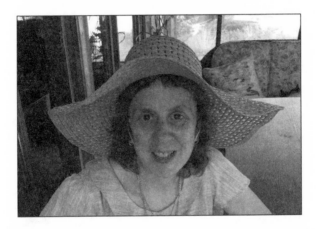

Ruth Lauer-Manenti has been teaching yoga for two decades to students from around the world, primarily at the Jivamukti Yoga School in New York City, her home. Ruth is the author of two previous books, *An Offering of Leaves* and *Sweeping the Dust*. Ruth also has an MFA from the Yale School of Art, where she later taught printmaking, and has also taught drawing and painting at Dartmouth College. She regularly exhibits her work.

ruthlauermanenti.com

ABOUT THE PUBLISHER

LANTERN BOOKS was founded in 1999 on the principle of living with a greater depth and commitment to the preservation of the natural world. In addition to publishing books on animal advocacy, vegetarianism, religion, and environmentalism, Lantern is dedicated to printing books in the U.S. on recycled paper and saving resources in day-to-day operations. Lantern is honored to be a recipient of the highest standard in environmentally responsible publishing from the Green Press Initiative.

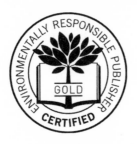

lanternbooks.com